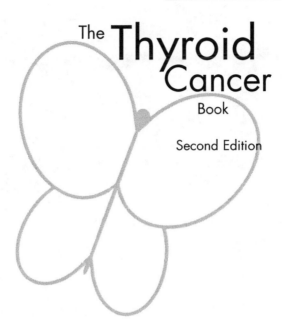

The Thyroid Cancer

Book

Second Edition

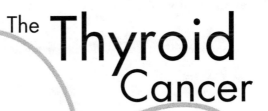

The Thyroid
Cancer
Book

Second Edition

M. Sara Rosenthal, Ph.D.

Author of *The Thyroid Sourcebook*,
recommended by the *New York Times*,
The Thyroid Sourcebook for Women, and
The Hypothyroid Sourcebook

First published in Canada in 2002 by
Your Health Press™, a division of Sarahealth, Inc.
in association with Trafford Publishing.

National Library of Canada Cataloguing in Publication

Rosenthal, M. Sara
    The thyroid cancer book / M. Sara Rosenthal.

Includes bibliographical references and index.
ISBN 1-55395-059-3

    1. Thyroid gland—Cancer—Popular works. I. Title.
RC280.T6R69 2002   616.99'444   C2002-904183-X

Your Health Press™
A division of Sarahealth, Inc.
Printed in Canada

IMPORTANT NOTICE:

The purpose of this book is to educate. It is sold with the understanding that the author and publisher shall have neither liability nor responsibility for any injury caused or alleged to be caused directly or indirectly by the information contained in this book. While every effort has been made to ensure its accuracy, the book's contents should not be construed as medical advice. Moreover, there is continuing controversy and debate amongst various thyroid cancer experts over management and treatment issues, and there is often no consensus amongst these experts as to the best approaches in various situations. Each person's health needs are unique. To obtain recommendations appropriate to your particular situation, please consult a qualified health care provider. The herbal remedies recommended in this book are for educational purposes only and should not be used without consulting a qualified expert in herbal medicine.

This book was published *on-demand* **in cooperation with Trafford Publishing.**
On-demand publishing is a unique process and service of making a book available for retail sale to the public taking advantage of on-demand manufacturing and Internet marketing.
On-demand publishing includes promotions, retail sales, manufacturing, order fulfilment, accounting and collecting royalties on behalf of the author.

Suite 6E, 2333 Government St., Victoria, B.C. V8T 4P4, CANADA

Phone	250-383-6864	Toll-free	1-888-232-4444 (Canada & US)
Fax	250-383-6804	E-mail	sales@trafford.com
Web site	www.trafford.com	TRAFFORD PUBLISHING IS A DIVISION OF TRAFFORD HOLDINGS LTD.	
Trafford Catalogue #02-0217		www.trafford.com/robots/02-0217.html	

10   9   8   7

Other Your Health Press™ Titles

Other Books on Thyroid Disease by M. Sara Rosenthal

The Thyroid Sourcebook, 4th edition (McGraw-Hill, 2000)
The Thyroid Sourcebook for Women (McGraw-Hill, 1999)
The Hypothyroid Sourcebook (McGraw-Hill, 2002)

Books on Other Health Topics by M. Sara Rosenthal

The Gynecological Sourcebook, 4th edition (McGraw-Hill, 2003)
(Published in Canada as *Gynecological Health* by Penguin Books).
The Pregnancy Sourcebook, 3rd edition (McGraw-Hill, 1999)
The Fertility Sourcebook, 3rd edition (McGraw-Hill, 2002)
The Breastfeeding Sourcebook, 3rd edition (McGraw-Hill, 2000)
The Breast Sourcebook, 2nd edition (McGraw-Hill, 1999)
The Gastrointestinal Sourcebook (McGraw-Hill, 1998)
The Type 2 Diabetic Woman (McGraw-Hill, 1999)
Women and Depression (McGraw-Hill, 2000)
Women of the '60s Turning 50 (Penguin Books, 2000)
Women and Passion (Penguin Books, 2000)
The Canadian Type 2 Diabetes Sourcebook (Wiley Canada, 2001)
Managing PMS Naturally (Penguin Books, 2002)
Women Managing Stress (Penguin Books, 2002)
Natural Woman's Guide to Living with the Complications of Diabetes
(2003, New Page Books)
Natural Woman's Guide to Hormone Replacement Therapy
(2003, New Page Books)
The Skinny on Fat (2004, McClelland & Stewart, Toronto)

50 Ways Series

50 Ways to Prevent Colon Cancer (McGraw-Hill, 2000)
50 Ways Women Can Prevent Heart Disease (McGraw-Hill, 2000)
50 Ways to Manage Heartburn and Reflux (McGraw-Hill, 2001)
50 Ways to Manage Type 2 Diabetes (McGraw-Hill, 2001)
50 Ways to Manage and Prevent Stress (McGraw-Hill, 2001)
50 Ways to Fight Depression Without Drugs (McGraw-Hill, 2001)

Recommended "Companion Books" for Thyroid Cancer Survivors

The Hypothyroid Sourcebook
Stopping Cancer at the Source
50 Ways to Manage and Prevent Stress
50 Ways to Fight Depression Without Drugs

Acknowledgments

This book would not have come to fruition without the meticulous medical review of chapters 1 through 7, and portions of the Introduction, by Kenneth B. Ain, M.D., Professor of Medicine, Director, Thyroid Oncology Section, Division of Hematology & Oncology, Department of Internal Medicine, University of Kentucky Medical Center, and Director, Thyroid Cancer Research Laboratory, Veterans Affairs Medical Center, Lexington, Kentucky. I am also greatly indebted to other endocrinologists who contributed comments to the first edition of this book, including Yolanda C. Oertel, M.D., Pathologist, Washington Hospital Center.

I'd like to thank the following people for their work and commitment on various editions of *The Thyroid Sourcebook*, which helped to lay so much of the groundwork for this book: Robert Volpe, M.D., F.R.C.P., F.A.C.P., who served as a past medical adviser; Daniel Drucker, M.D., F.R.C.P.; Heather Dawson, M.D., F.R.C.P., F.A.C.P.; Gillian Arsenault, M.D., F.R.C.P.; Susan George, M.D., F.R.C.P., F.A.C.P.; Leslie Goldenberg, M.D., F.R.C.P.; Matthew Lazar, F.R.C.P., F.A.C.P. and Irving B. Rosen, M.D., F.R.C.S., F.A.C.S.

I'd also like to thank members of both the Thyroid Cancer Survivor's Association and the Canadian Thyroid Cancer Support Group (Thry'vors) Inc. for their suggestions for content.

Finally, this book would not have made it into your hands were it not for Larissa Kostoff, Editorial Director of Your Health Press™, and Laura Tulchinsky, Marketing Director of Your Health Press™.

CONTENTS

Discover Your Life Force Energy
Pressure Point Therapies
Aromatherapy
Qi Gong
Feng Shui
Meditation
Calm Your Nerves
Counseling

INTRODUCTION

Many of you reading this book already know parts of my story, which I have revealed in past works on thyroid disease, such as *The Thyroid Sourcebook*, first published in 1993 (now in its fourth edition). I was diagnosed with thyroid cancer in 1983, at the age of 20. (Okay—now you know my age!) All I heard was "cancer;" I had no idea what a thyroid gland was. The product of a broken home, a bitter custody battle and a "deadbeat Dad" who refused to pay child support despite ample means, I was living with my mother, who was trying to make ends meet on a secretary's salary. We hovered above the poverty line in 1983; I was in second year university and planned to apply to law school (even though I was really a writer). My dream at that time was to go into family law so I could represent children who, like myself, were torn apart in custody battles. I never wrote my L-SAT. Instead, I got thyroid cancer and my whole world changed. But the goal of turning my "lemons" into lemonade was still met—just in an entirely different way than I planned.

Had I lived in the United States, my mother would not have had the money to pay for the medical treatment I needed, and probably would not have had adequate insurance coverage. In Canada, I was covered under my provincial health care. At the time my cancer was diagnosed, it had spread throughout my neck, and was in a secondary stage. I had a total thyroidectomy (removal of the thyroid gland) and neck dissection (removal of cancerous lymph nodes), followed by a 100 millicurie dose of radioactive iodine—the maximum allowable dose in my hospital at that time. Depressed and hypothyroid, I dragged around my university campus, and prepared for various scans. The last part of my treatment entailed taking the bus everyday for a month to the bowels of the hospital for my external radiation therapy treatments, which made me sicker than any of the previous treatments. As I sit here pushing 40, I'm amazed I went through this experience with almost no information about what cancer was or what a thyroid gland was. When the fourth year medical student on duty during my thyroid surgery asked me out on a date (after I had gone home), I accepted because I saw it as an opportunity to get some information. In essence, I dated my way to thyroid cancer information because it was the only way I could get it. In fact, I suffered more from a lack of information about thyroid cancer than from the actual cancer itself. This is the book I wish I had when I was first diagnosed, and it is also the book I need now, as a long-time survivor of thyroid cancer.

What I thought at the time was a lot of information about my cancer from my head and neck surgeon would sound today like *See Spot Run*. Now, having completed my doctorate in bioethics (also called medical ethics), I can't believe what I wasn't told. And I have spoken in public about the inept handling of my biopsy procedure, an older procedure not done anymore in which the initial "lump" was removed in its entirety. (I wasn't given any pain medication, nor was I given enough local anesthetic, and told that it was such a "simple" procedure that there was no need to bring anyone to the hospital with me.) When I cried in pain, the tanned plastic surgeon biopsying the lump actually yelled at me, yet he was not at all the appropriate person to do the procedure. (I was referred to him by my family doctor when I insisted on having the lump removed—something my family doctor didn't think was necessary.) Incredibly, when the lump was found to be cancerous, no one told me about it. Instead, my doctor called my mother and told *her* about my cancer. And so it was *she* who told me the news, in the absence of any physician. She could barely explain it to me properly, and for the first several minutes of that discussion, I thought it was *she* who had cancer. From both the lay and academic perspectives, this was an outrageous way for a doctor—even in 1983—to handle the cancer diagnosis of a 20-year-old woman.

I have seen thyroid cancer go from an unheard-of cancer that barely received a paragraph of note in most cancer books or materials put out by cancer organizations to a commonly diagnosed cancer inspiring large support networks, including the recently formed Thyroid Cancer Survivor's Association (*www.thyca.org*) and Thry'vors (*http://groups.yahoo.com/group/Thryvors/join*), a Canadian organization of thyroid cancer survivors. When I wrote the first non-technical consumer book on thyroid disease, *The Thyroid Sourcebook*, I never imagined that there would be enough of an audience to warrant a separate book on thyroid cancer. For many years, the chapter I included in *The Thyroid Sourcebook* on thyroid cancer was the only accessible information that thyroid cancer patients could turn to. I became convinced in the later 1990s that a separate thyroid cancer book ought to be written, but no one would publish it because thyroid cancer remained a "rare" cancer. Essentially, that means no mainstream publisher could justify spending the money on a book geared towards what's still considered a small market. In 2000, when I launched my health promotion company and website (*sarahealth.com*), I had a vision of creating a health publishing company that would service the needs of people suffering from rare or stigmatizing health problems— health problems about which little or nothing is written. What followed was the birth of a series of books by Your Health Press™, which are dedicated to orphan diseases such as thyroid cancer, as well as controversial or stigmatizing health issues. As of this writing, this is the first thyroid cancer book written for the consumer by a thyroid cancer survivor. It's designed as a complete and comprehensive resource for thyroid cancer survivors. But before you move on to other chapters, there are two things you need to know before you can put it all together. You need to understand what a thyroid gland does in the body, and you need to understand what cancer does in the body.

What Is a Thyroid Gland?

Many of you reading this book probably have other general books on thyroid disease, which may include past books of mine, such as *The Thyroid Sourcebook*. However, to save you some time, the following is a brief primer on what the thyroid gland does all day in your body.

The "thyroid" was named in the 1600s. The word itself is Greek for "shield," because of its butterfly shape. Your thyroid gland is located in the lower part of your neck, in front of your windpipe, and it produces two thyroid hormones: thyroxine, known as T4 (four iodine atoms), and triiodothyronine, known as T3 (three iodine atoms). Thyroid hormone (the two hormones are referred to in the singular; the word "hormone" is Greek for "stimulator") is then secreted into the circulatory system and becomes widely distributed throughout the body. It's one of the basic regulators of the functions of every cell and every tissue within the body, and a steady supply is crucial for good health. In essence, your thyroid affects you from head to toe—including skin and hair!

If you were to break down exactly how much T4 and T3 is secreted by your thyroid, you'd find that 90 percent of the thyroid output is T4, and only 10 percent is T3. Although these hormones have the same effect in your body, T4 must be converted into T3 before it is able to affect the body. T4 turns into T3 by shedding an iodine atom, a process that is regulated differently by different body parts.

Iodine

Your thyroid gland extracts iodine from various foods, including certain vegetables, shell fish, milk products (cow udders are washed with large amounts of iodine, which wind up in your milk) and *anything* with iodized salt. Normally, we take in sufficient iodine through our diet. Our thyroids are very sensitive to iodine. When the thyroid gland isn't able to obtain sufficient quantities of iodine, it can enlarge and you develop what's called a goiter. It can also become over or underactive. (See *The Thyroid Sourcebook* for more on goiters, iodine deficiency, hyperthyroidism and hypothyroidism.)

The Pituitary Gland

The pituitary gland (often referred to as the "master gland") is situated at the base of the skull and regularly monitors T4 and T3 "stock" in your body's blood levels. When stock is low, it sends a message to your thyroid gland—in the form of a stimulating hormone called TSH (thyroid stimulating hormone)—and orders it to produce more. The pituitary gland secretes increased amounts of TSH when T4 and/or T3 levels are low. That's why the TSH test is so telling: when your TSH level is high, it's a sign that you're hypothyroid; when it's low, it is a sign that you're hyperthyroid. As a thyroid cancer survivor, the TSH test will help you know whether your thyroid medication is adequate. This is discussed more in chapter 7.

The Role of Calcitonin

Your thyroid gland rents space to additional thyroid cells called C cells, which make the hormone calcitonin and do not make thyroid hormone. This hormone helps to regulate calcium, and hence helps to prevent osteoporosis. But to your *bones*, calcitonin is kind of like a tonsil; it serves a useful purpose, but when the hormone isn't manufactured, due to the absence of a thyroid gland (if it's removed or ablated by radioactive iodine), you won't really notice any effects, just as you don't miss your tonsils. Calcium levels are really controlled by the parathyroid glands, discussed further on. (Women need to be aware that the hormone estrogen also influences calcium levels, which is why after menopause, osteoporosis is such a concern. (See *The Thyroid Sourcebook for Women* for more on this.)

Calcitonin comes into play when screening for a rare type of thyroid cancer called medullary thyroid cancer, which is sometimes genetic in origin and which is discussed in detail in chapter 4.

The Role of Thyroglobulin

Although this sounds like a Halloween candy, thyroglobulin is a specific protein made only by your thyroid cells, used mostly by the thyroid gland itself to make and store thyroid hormone. Like calcitonin, this substance isn't all that important to your body once your thyroid is gone; you won't miss it. The only role thyroglobulin plays is in screening for thyroid cancer recurrence (normally, produced by thyroid cells and thyroid cancer cells it leaks into blood where it can be measured). This is discussed more in chapter 7.

What is Cancer?

Now that you know what the thyroid gland does, it's also useful to understand in more general terms, what "cancer" actually means. Cancer is the general term for the abnormal growth of cells. When the abnormal cell reproduces, it has the ability to invade or metastasize to other parts of the body. The actual word "cancer" is Latin for crab. It was, in fact, the crab-like appearance of tumors that inspired the Roman physician Galen to actually name cancer. In Greek, "karkinos" originally meant "crab" too, which is how Hippocrates first identified and classified this illness 2,500 years ago.

Cancer was rarely noted in the ancient world, and is not mentioned at all in the Bible or the *Yellow Emperor's Classic of Internal Medicine,* the ancient medicine book of China. It began to be diagnosed more extensively around the time of the Industrial Revolution.

The cancer cell frequently destroys the organ from which it originates. As it spreads into various parts of the body, it interferes with the jobs of regular cells, confuses other organs, and can wreak havoc. It's basically a terrorist cell, hijacking surrounding organs and other cells. Cancer cells use the lymph system or blood vessels to get into the bloodstream and then travel throughout the body. These cells love organs that have multiple blood vessels and nutrients, such as bones, lungs, and brains— common areas where cancer spreads.

Cancer cells are classified into four main groups: carcinoma, sarcoma, leukemia and lymphoma. A carcinoma refers to cancerous cells coming from epithelial cells – cells that line various organs. You'll find carcinomas in organs that tend to secrete something (milk, mucus, digestive juices, and so on). Common sites for carcinomas are breasts, lungs, and colons. Carcinomas account for 80 to 90 percent of all human cancers, and are generally slow-growing. There is always a prefix attached to the word "carcinoma" that will tell us where the carcinoma is growing, and the kinds of cells that are involved. An adenocarcinoma, for example, is a carcinoma starting in glandular cells. When you just see the word "oma" by itself, it means tumor. An adenoma refers to a clump of benign glandular cells; a fibroma refers to a clump of benign fibrous cells, and so on. When the cells are malignant, the word carcinoma is attached to the end, as in adenocarcinoma. When it comes to thyroid tumors, benign tumors are more frequent than adenocarcinomas, which are malignant. It gets even more specific. You'll need to know where the adenocarcinoma itself originated. Think of it like this: carcinoma used by itself is as descriptive as saying "sweater." Adenocarcinoma is like saying "wool sweater." More specific descriptions can be "lambswool sweater" or "angora sweater." And there can be other prefixes that are synonymous with saying "blue angora sweater." There are literally hundreds of carcinomas, all described by a different combination of prefixes that identify the parts of the bodies involved, the shape of the carcinomas, etc.

Sarcomas are cancerous cells coming from supporting connective tissue. Sarcomas are rare and account for only two percent of all human cancers, but tend to be more aggressive than carcinomas. Again, the prefixes before the word tell you where the sarcoma is located, what it's made of, what shape it is, etc., while sometimes sarcomas are named after the doctors who discovered them. The difference between a carcinoma and a sarcoma is equal to the difference between a sweater and a boot; both are different things, but related. Nonetheless, both have different physical properties, are made of different materials, available in different colors, and so on.

Since cancer cells are living cells, it's in their nature to continue to live. So the first thing cancer cells do is grow; they grow at a faster rate than normal cells. They'll simply begin growing where they first originated, be it in the thyroid, lung, or colon. Then they mutate from the other cells that surround them. After they get to a certain age, they want to move out and leave their original nest. So they spread out into surrounding fat and tissue.

A very crucial need of the cancer cell is to eat. So the cancer cell sends out protein messengers (called tumor angiogenesis factors) that create new blood vessels to feed it. If a cancer cell can manage to grow, spread and eat, it will live, and we'll experience the result of this in the form of a tumor. If any of these functions is stopped, the cancer will die. As you've guessed by now, treatments will therefore attempt to interfere with these functions. These treatments aim to: stop the cells from growing; stop the cells from changing or mutating; stop the cells from spreading; or stop the cells from eating.

If the cancer continues to live, it will simply continue these same basic behaviors: it will grow bigger; change and mutate even more to trick the immune system; and spread out even more by bursting into surrounding structures and into the blood vessels. Finally, if the cells reach adulthood, they'll want to settle down and find a good home, preferably an organ rich in blood vessels, like liver, lungs, and bone. So the cells attach to these blood vessels, and pass through them into such an organ. And they'll continue to make themselves comfortable so that they can reproduce more and more. This means setting themselves up with a new blood supply to make the organ more conducive to their growth. And so it goes, until the cancer occupies many sites in the body. The most important thing to remember is that none of this happens immediately; it can take years for these cancer cells to really spread.

Differentiated vs. Undifferentiated

Cancer cells are classified into two behavioral categories: differentiated and undifferentiated. These terms refer to the degree of maturation of the cancer cells. Differentiated cancer cells resemble the more normal cells of their origin. A differentiated cancer cell that originates in the thyroid, for example, would look and act more like a normal thyroid cell. In fact, these differentiated cancer cells do not reproduce as rapidly as undifferentiated cells. Differentiated cancer cells look different under the microscope from undifferentiated cancer cells; they also have structural differences that allow doctors to tell the type of cancer cell, and therefore predict how rapidly the cell is growing, and the degree of malignancy. But both differentiated and undifferentiated cells are often treatable; key factors are tumor size and lymph node status. Often, you won't find a purely differentiated cell. It may look just moderately abnormal. Because of this, there are sub-classifications: moderately differentiated, well differentiated, or poorly differentiated. These classifications are known as the cells' *grading*. A high grade means that the cell is immature, looks wilder or poorly differentiated and therefore faster growing; a low-grade cancer cell is mature, looks more normal or well-differentiated, slow-growing, and less aggressive. However, this is a terribly basic explanation of cell grading, something that has far more complex criteria.

Undifferentiated cancer is made up of very primitive cells that look wild and untamed, bearing little or no resemblance to the cells of origin. This is more dangerous because the cells may then spread faster. There are cases, though, when undifferentiated cancer isn't very aggressive, despite the fact that it involves more primitive cells. In these cases, the cancer looks wilder than it behaves. This is often the case in breast cancers.

There are also mixes of these different cells, which affect the aggressiveness of the disease. For example, there can be mostly differentiated cells mixed in with a few undifferentiated cells, or vice versa. Whatever is most aggressive will affect the behavior of the cancer; mostly differentiated cells will slow down whatever undifferentiated cells exist, while mostly undifferentiated cells will speed up whatever differentiated cells exist.

Some differentiated cancers may evolve or mutate into more aggressive, rapidly growing undifferentiated cancers. This happens either because the differentiated cancer cell mutates, or because the wilder cells within the tumor outgrow the more normal, differentiated cancer cells. This will then change the behavior of the tumor in later stages.

Okay—you're armed with the basics. Now you're ready to move on to the complex world of thyroid cancer.

1
WHO GETS THYROID CANCER?

In the early 1980s, the Emmy award-winning show *Lou Grant*, a spinoff from the old *Mary Tyler Moore Show* (which I worshipped) actually did an episode about thyroid cancer! I kid you not. In this episode, Lou Grant (who, in this spinoff, is now a news editor for a major Los Angeles daily) feels a lump in his neck while shaving, and is diagnosed with thyroid cancer. The episode shows his surgeon explaining what the thyroid gland is, how it uses iodine and how radioactive iodine is used to treat thyroid cancer. I almost fell off my chair in the early 1990s when I saw this episode in a rerun. It was terribly ironic for me, considering that my own thyroid cancer was diagnosed just a few months after that original episode aired. The *Lou Grant* show was canceled by CBS after a couple of seasons because it was considered too controversial for its time; the thyroid cancer episode remains testament to just *how* ahead of its time the show really was.

By all accounts, thyroid cancer is still considered a rare cancer, accounting for two percent of all cancers. It was almost unheard of by the average person in the early 1980s; today, it's still rare enough to be a topic that mainstream publishers refuse to cover, due to such low numbers and a perceived poor market. Throughout the mid- to late 1990s, my book proposals for thyroid cancer were consistently rejected. But actually, thyroid cancer is now the fastest growing cancer, according to studies tracking cancer incidence (based on the number of cases per 100,000 people per year). Thyroid cancer was seen to increase at a steady rate of 6.6 percent among women and 4.2 percent among men per year. In 2001, there were 19,500 new cases of thyroid cancer in the United States, and about 1,300 deaths, according to the latest statistics available from the

American Cancer Society. In fact more people were diagnosed with thyroid cancer in 2001 than those with liver or brain cancer, which demonstrates that thyroid cancer ought to be considered a common cancer today. At the 2003 American Thyroid Association conference, thyroid cancer was ranked as the fastest rising cancer in women, topping lung and breast cancers. Women outnumber men in developing thyroid cancer by three to one. Put another way, women account for 77 percent of all new cases of thyroid cancer, and 61 percent of all deaths from thyroid cancer occur in women. In 2001, 4,600 men developed thyroid cancer, compared to 15,000 women; 500 deaths from thyroid cancer occurred in men, and 800 deaths occurred in women. This statistical imbalance may have something to do with the fact that thyroid problems are seen roughly 10 times more frequently in women, which I discuss more in *The Thyroid Sourcebook for Women*.

The Fallout Story

If you follow the wind patterns from nuclear testing fallout, nuclear facilities, or even buried nuclear waste (which we may not even know about), you'll find a trail of thyroid cancer. The most common known cause of thyroid cancer is exposure to radioactive iodine, which affects the cells of the thyroid gland, causing them to mutate. I was born in Winnipeg, Manitoba, Canada, which is considered the geographic centre of North America, just downwind from Nevada. A 14-year National Cancer Institute study, published in 1997, looked at the health risks of radioactive fallout released at the Nevada Test Site from 1951 through 1958. The study concluded that people living in the midwestern regions of North America were more at risk for thyroid cancer, particularly if they were children during the testing. (The producers of the *Lou Grant* show probably didn't realize how accurate they were when writing their thyroid cancer script, as Lou Grant was supposedly born and bred in Minneapolis, Minnesota, where the fictitious WJM newsroom originated on the old *Mary Tyler Moore Show*.)

Radioactive iodine is emitted whenever fallout from nuclear accidents, testing and, of course, atomic bombs occurs. Most unfortunately, we're seeing a tremendous increase in childhood thyroid cancer in certain "hot" areas, such as parts of Russia, Belarus, and the Ukraine exposed to fallout from the 1986 Chernobyl nuclear reactor accident, which released 40 million curies of radioactive iodine into the atmosphere. That's a lot, considering that thyroid cancer patients typically receive 100 millicuries, discussed in chapter 6.

Reports of high rates of thyroid cancer are also coming in from Hanford, Washington, where residents were exposed to fallout from the Hanford nuclear facility, which produced plutonium for nuclear weapons from 1944 through 1957.

Anyone living downwind from the Nevada Test Site (residents in southwestern Utah for example), between the years 1951 and 1962 is also vulnerable to thyroid cancer.

Other areas affected by fallout are the Marshall Islands in the South Pacific, as a result of atomic bomb testing at Bikini Atoll in 1954. Here, thyroid cancer occurs 100 times more frequently than in the general population.

In the aftermath of a very long Cold War, more information is slowly becoming available about just how "hot" North America, Europe and other parts of the world really are. The predictions are that thyroid cancer incidence will continue to rise in our lifetimes. But we're seeing this trend with a variety of other cancers, too. As far back as 1994, however, the North Dakota State Health Department reported that the incidence of thyroid cancer in that state had doubled from five to 10 percent. The increase was attributed to radioactive iodine fallout. The Oak Ridge Health Agreement Steering Panel reported that young women born in 1952 who drank contaminated milk from test fallout were more likely to develop thyroid cancer in their lifetimes than women born in the northeastern United States. The Energy Research Foundation in the U.S. concludes that there may be thousands of North Americans who ingested milk that was contaminated with this fallout, and who, as a result, are at greater risk for thyroid cancer.

Thyroid cancer may not be the only consequence of radioactive fallout. For example, a daily newspaper called the *Tennessean* published an investigatory report on the "mysterious" thyroid diseases in the late 1990s that afflicted people working at and living near nuclear weapons plants and research facilities from California to New York. Not only was there a high incidence of thyroid cancer found, but also a high incidence of autoimmune thyroid diseases. And those working at and living near nuclear facilities in Tennessee, Ohio, Kentucky, Colorado, South Carolina, New Mexico, Idaho, New York, California, Texas and Washington State all reported the same illness trend.

The nuclear accident at the Chernobyl atomic power station on April 26, 1986 exposed millions of people with healthy thyroid glands to excessive levels of radioactive iodine. People living within a 30 km zone of the accident inhaled the radioactive iodine, while people living outside the 30 km zone ingested the radioactive iodine. For reasons not quite understood, potassium iodide tablets (thyroid blocking agents) weren't distributed to the public by the appropriate government agencies, except in Poland. Now, there appears to be an eightyfold increase in the incidence of thyroid cancer in children, and an increase of thyroid cancer in adults in Belarus, Russia,and the Ukraine. For example, one study out of the Ukraine found that between 1981 and 1985, the number of new cases of thyroid cancer in children 0 to 14 totaled 25. But between 1986 and 1994, the number of new cases of thyroid cancer in this age group totaled 210, with peak periods in 1992 and 1993. Without a doubt the most infamous nuclear reactor accident was Chernobyl in 1986. Since then, another major nuclear reactor accident took place on September 29, 1999 in Tokaimura, Japan. Residents in the area were told to stay indoors with windows and vents closed in order to minimize exposure to various radioactive gases that were released. In the case of Tokaimura, radioactive iodine was released in small quantities into the air for a full week before the reactor problem was detected. By October 8, 1999, the levels of radioactive iodine released into the air were twice the allowable levels.

The fallout story makes sense once you understand how the thyroid gland works (see Introduction), and that it needs to extract iodine from various sources—because iodine is the building block it needs to make thyroid hormone. Thyroid hormone is also the building block *we* need to function properly. So, the thyroid gland has a sort of fatal attraction to iodine and radioactive iodine, which has the unique ability to head straight for the thyroid gland. There is some debate over whether breast cancer is related to radioactive iodine, too, but this is discussed more in chapter 6. The bottom line is this: radioactive iodine causes changes in the DNA of your healthy thyroid cells. Ironically, radioactive iodine can also be used to target and "kill" cancerous thyroid cells. See chapter 6 for more information on the radioactive iodine story.

The X-Ray Story

In other cases, radiation to the head and neck area from high-dose x-rays (common from the 1940s through the 1970s) during childhood or adolescence can cause thyroid cancer to develop later in life. In the 1940s and 1950s, x-ray therapy was commonly used to treat infants with enlarged thymus glands (which were falsely believed to cause crib death) and children with enlarged adenoids and tonsils. X-ray therapy was also used to treat facial acne in teenagers, birthmarks, whooping cough, scalp ringworm, and sometimes as a means to improve hearing for the deaf. The practice of using x-rays began in the 1920s, peaked in the 1940s and 1950s, and then slowly petered out by the 1960s. The treatment was administered in one of two ways. One way involved an x-ray machine (called external beam radiation); the other way involved placing radioactive material like radium directly in or on the tissue to be treated. The immediate results were often promising. For example, acne improved while acne scarring was reduced, and some forms of deafness were improved. (Enlarged lymph tissue would sometimes block the inner ear and cause deafness; radiation was used to shrink the lymph tissue and improve hearing.)

However, the long-term consequences of x-ray treatment canceled out any short-term benefits. Unlike laser treatments, X-ray treatments weren't concentrated onto one small area and irradiated surrounding areas. Since the thyroid gland is located in the center of the neck, x-rays beamed at the face (to treat acne), chest (to treat asthma, pneumonia, and even hyperthyroidism), adenoids, tonsils, thymus gland, ears, or scalp were also targeting the thyroid gland. By the 1950s, doctors began to notice an increase in benign and malignant nodules on the thyroid glands of patients who had previously been treated with x-rays. Then, by the late 1950s and early 1960s, it was found that many victims of the atomic bomb in Hiroshima and Nagasaki were developing malignant tumors on their thyroid glands.

X-rays were also widely used in the 1930s and 1940s to determine fetal positions in prenatal care. This was known as pelvimetry, and unfortunately exposed the fetal tissue to radiation. Let's also not forget the radiation used to treat congenital heart problems, as well as those standard TB exams most employers demanded between 1920 and 1960. Much of the radiation therapy between the 1920s and 1960s was probably poorly documented, meaning that there was more exposure than was recorded.

Thyroid cancer is not the only cancer caused by exposure to x-rays. In his controversial book *Preventing Breast Cancer: The Story of a Major, Proven, Preventable Cause of This Disease* (1995), John W. Gofman, M.D., Ph.D. concludes that about 75 percent of breast cancer cases are largely due to past medical-related radiation.

It's estimated that millions of people throughout North America, Europe and the U.K. received these treatments in the past. (In the U.S., over two million people alone are estimated to have received them.) Generally, benign thyroid lumps (a.k.a. "nodules") and thyroid cancer have been discovered in people anywhere from 10 to 60 years following x-ray therapy.

It's important to note that not all people exposed to radiation develop thyroid cancer. Thyroid cancer experts maintain that "most" people who are diagnosed with thyroid cancer have no "known" exposure to radiation. But as the author of *Stopping Cancer At the Source*, a book on environmental causes of cancer, I can reasonably say that all of us living in this toxic soup called Earth have been exposed to countless carcinogens (meaning cancer-causing agents) if we were born after 1945. The fact that some of these carcinogens trip our "cancer genes" or oncogenes is how genetics may play a role in thyroid cancer.

The Gene Story

There is only one type of thyroid cancer that's sometimes known to be absolutely genetic in the absence of an external or environmental trigger: this is called *medullary thyroid cancer*, and I discuss it in detail in chapter 4. But there are also certain types of thyroid cancers that are believed to have a hereditary link. Thyroid cancer falls under the general category of "endocrine" cancers, and some researchers believe that people who come from a family where other endocrine cancers (such as ovarian or adrenal) seem to strike, may be particularly vulnerable to thyroid cancers. In addition some genetic syndromes associated with colon polyps also have papillary thyroid cancers and new studies show family clusters of this cancer.

Is There a Thyroid Cancer Gene?

To date, we don't know of a "thyroid cancer gene" that absolutely predicts thyroid cancer, other than the gene causing inherited medullary thyroid cancer, which is quite distinct from the more common types of thyroid cancer, explained in chapter 3. We are living in an age, however, where other types of cancer genes are being found, such as breast cancer genes and colon cancer genes. In these cases, finding a cancer gene is not necessarily meaningful information, since there's a wide range of varied effects of these genes in causing cancer. And frequently, there is nothing one can do to reasonably prevent the cancer for which the gene is a marker, although lifestyle changes can help to prevent certain cancers. For example, lung cancer, which tops the charts, would be almost completely eradicated if people stopped smoking—even if they were genetically wired for it. Additionally, many cancers are triggered by environmental factors, which turn on various genes. That's how it normally works.

But the gene for inherited medullary thyroid cancer is different. This is one of the few cases when having the gene almost guarantees that you will develop inherited medullary thyroid cancer, discussed more in chapter 4. In this case, genetic screening can be a useful tool in predicting who may develop this type of thyroid cancer because it can also be used to prevent this type of cancer (someone who tests positive for the gene will have a total thyroidectomy, thus removing the threat). If you or someone in your family has had medullary thyroid cancer, it's recommended that the person being treated for thyroid cancer see a genetic counselor to discuss the benefits of screening for this disease to prevent cancer in the rest of the family.

A wider issue surrounding genetic screening is the fast-approaching future—a future where a long list of genetic information may be compiled about each person from birth. In some cases, diseases that are stigmatizing could affect one's social status. Genetic testing can also reveal paternity, which may also be socially stigmatizing. In the case of inherited medullary thyroid cancer, genetic screening is considered to be more beneficial than harmful for two reasons:

1. Since having this particular gene almost always means that medullary thyroid cancer, which can be very aggressive, will develop, removing the thyroid gland in a person who tests positive for the gene can prevent a real, predictable life-threatening disease. Again, unlike other cancers, we can not only predict who will get inherited medullary thyroid cancer, but we can actually prevent it.

2. Thyroid cancer is not a socially stigmatizing disease in the same way that diseases such as AIDS may be stigmatizing; therefore, knowing that you have a thyroid cancer gene will probably not affect employment, or social interactions.

For more information on genetic screening for inherited medullary thyroid cancer, see chapter 4.

Signs of Thyroid Cancer

It's important to recognize the signs of thyroid cancer, particularly if your thyroid has been exposed to radiation. Often the signs are not that obvious, but they can include:

- A hard and painless lump (also called nodule) anywhere on your neck.
- A thyroid nodule that continues to enlarge.
- Difficulty swallowing food or liquids.
- Change in your voice or hoarseness (this may indicate that the cancer is spreading beyond the thyroid gland).
- Pain in your neck tissues, jawbone, or ear (this is a very uncommon sign of thyroid cancer but has been reported).
- A diagnosis of "sleep apnea," which has come on suddenly (this is a sleep disorder characterized by interrupted breathing). This is very rare, but there have been cases where thyroid cancer patients have been *falsely* diagnosed with sleep apnea when, in fact, a growing thyroid tumor was present. In these cases, difficulties with breathing were actually caused by a spreading thyroid tumor, which can block breathing passages!

In the great majority of people with thyroid cancer, the first sign of cancer is a non-tender lump in the neck that is found by themselves, a relative, or a doctor during a routine exam. The signs of medullary thyroid cancer, as well as anaplastic thyroid cancer are somewhat different and are discussed separately in chapters 4 and 5.

The "Good Cancer"

Since the 1940s, the most common types of thyroid cancer (papillary, follicular or a mix of the two) have been completely treatable 95 percent of the time. The reason is that papillary and follicular thyroid cancers grow relatively slowly, compared to other kinds of cancers, such as colon, prostate, or breast. In essence, most types of thyroid cancers take a very long time to spread. In fact, you could conceivably walk around with undiagnosed thyroid cancer for a decade and still respond well to treatment. Second, radioactive iodine (discovered in the 1940s) can often eradicate and/or control the growth of thyroid cancer. In a way, radioactive iodine is close to a "miracle cure" for thyroid cancer. So the first thing most people diagnosed with thyroid cancer hear is: "This is a good cancer." But because it's "a good cancer," there has been an assumption that thyroid cancer patients do not suffer and do not need the same level of psychosocial support as other cancer patients. Thyroid cancer patients go through a great deal of treatment to become cancer free—and remain cancer free. So hearing that you've got a "good cancer" is not that comforting when you're struggling to fight cancer. I've provided a rich array of information in chapter 8 on emotional and spiritual healing, because most thyroid cancer patients don't feel that knowing they have "good cancer" substitutes for the psychosocial support they need. I've also provided information on self-healing and complementary medicine in chapter 9.

The "good cancer" line is also deceiving, especially when we know that some people *do* die from thyroid cancer, particularly those who are diagnosed with a rare form of thyroid cancer known as anaplastic thyroid cancer (see chapter 5). Also, in some cases, well-differentiated thyroid cancers can become more aggressive or poorly differentiated with time, which has to do with the biology of the tumor changes.

The majority of the thyroid cancer stories go like this: the thyroid cancer is usually caught in a primary or secondary stage. In the primary stage, a malignant nodule or lump is found on the thyroid gland; in the secondary stage, a malignant nodule is found somewhere on the neck, invading surrounding tissues, or in a lymph node nearby, which is traced to the thyroid gland. Therefore, in a secondary stage, the thyroid cancer has already spread beyond the thyroid gland. Thyroid cancer can also spread into the lungs and bone, but this is more unusual than usual. For more details, see chapters 3 through 5. Essentially, it's misleading to call thyroid cancer a "good cancer" when it's a type of cancer demonstrating the full range of behaviour, from slow growing, treatable cancers to one of the most aggressive types of cancers known (anaplastic thyroid cancer).

Can You Prevent Thyroid Cancer?

We can only prevent thyroid cancers that are directly caused by radioactive fallout. There's a blocking agent known as potassium iodide that can prevent radioactive iodine from being absorbed by the thyroid gland. This is the only specific way to protect against thyroid cancer triggered by radioactive iodine fallout; potassium iodide has no protective effect against any other kind of radiation. In this age of terrorism, people are nervous about potential nuclear terrorism, and potassium iodide is available through pharmacies. However, if a nuclear attack occurs, thyroid cancer would, of course, be the least of your worries. To be effective, potassium iodide must be dispensed just prior to being exposed to radioactive iodine, and then continued for the duration of the exposure. This is pretty difficult to do unless an accident or incident is predicted in advance, or the air path of a specific accident is tracked and therefore anticipated. And potassium iodide is not designed as a long-term therapy because of side effects that occur with prolonged use. Complications include serious allergic reactions, skin rashes, and thyroid disorders (like hypothyroidism or hyperthyroidism). In pregnant women, long-term use of potassium iodide can also cause the fetus to develop a goiter.

For the last 40 years, various government agencies around the world have monitored the amount of radioactive iodine in the air. And for many years, they've detected low levels of radioactive iodine fallout as a result of nuclear testing or reactor problems. Emergency plans for potassium iodide distribution in European countries require pills or tablets to be pre-distributed to households within three miles of nuclear plants, and possibly to households within six miles. Tablets also are to be stored at central locations, such as schools, factories and town halls, for quick distribution within 15.5 miles of plants. Since 1982, households within about nine miles of four nuclear plants have received tablets. Every five years, regional authorities repeat the distribution, to approximately 50,000 households, through the mail.

Distribution of potassium iodide in the United States remains controversial, but is being revisited in light of 9/11. To date, the Three Mile Island accident was the most serious nuclear reactor accident to have occurred in North America. Twenty years later, state and federal officials are still debating potassium iodide's costs and benefits. After the accident, a presidential commission strongly recommended stockpiling the drug near all U.S. reactor sites, but it was subsequently found that the average population exposure from radioactive iodine following Three Mile Island was very small—much less radiation than a chest x-ray, and thousands of times less than a routine diagnostic I131 uptake test. Because of these findings, and the possible effects of radioactive iodine, both the American and Canadian Food and Drug administrations haven't released potassium iodide as a drug for thyroid blocking, except to state/province and local governments who stockpile it for emergency use.

Even then, access is limited. The U.S. Nuclear Regulatory Commission (NRC) at one point endorsed stockpiling potassium iodide for any state that wanted it, but then reversed this decision because of budget concerns. When the NRC approached the Federal Emergency Management Agency (FEMA) to cover the costs of stockpiling potassium iodide, FEMA would not. So, many residents are now living in states with no stockpiles (or access to) potassium iodide, which would protect them from thyroid cancer in the event of a nuclear accident. As of this writing, Tennessee, Alabama, Arizona, Maine, California, and Ohio have a potassium iodide "stash" for the areas around and downwind from nuclear power plants. See Table 1.1 for a list of nuclear power plants.

The information spin about the Chernobyl accident was that despite the very large amounts of radioactive material that came from the Russian plant, only those working in and around the plant were exposed to any serious danger. Now we are seeing a thyroid cancer epidemic in that area, and a rise in many other cancers. The Chernobyl accident released 40 million curies of radioactive iodine into the atmosphere, exposing millions of people to excessive levels of radioactive iodine. People living within 30 kilometres of the accident inhaled the radioactive iodine, and people living outside this radius were also exposed to the substance. The incidence of thyroid cancer in children in Belarus, Russia, and the Ukraine appears to have increased more than eightyfold as a result of exposure. A Ukraine study reports that between 1981 and 1985, the number of new cases of thyroid cancer in children up to age 14 totaled 25. But between 1986 and 1994, the number of new cases of thyroid cancer in this age group totaled 210, peaking in 1992 and 1993.

For the best information on nuclear fallout exposure and thyroid cancer, see *http://thyroid.about.com/cs/nuclearexposure*. This is the website that Mary J. Shomon, runs. (The link to the National Institutes of Health "Fallout Report" is particularly useful!)

Reducing Radiation Risks

In order to control the cancer risks associated with hazardous levels of radiation, and to start identifying where unrecognized hazards from exposure might occur, experts recommend:

- Developing an inventory of sources of radioactive substances in Canada and the United States.
- Investigating how radioactive substances travel through the food chain.
- Imposing "chemical control rules" for suspected radioactive contaminants, which would result in more stringent standards.
- Studying radioactive emissions from energy production plants.

• Investigating ways of phasing out these materials wherever an increased cancer risk is found.

Nuclear Reactors

If you live in one of these states, you live near a nuclear reactor. And that means if there's an accident, you're at an increased risk of developing thyroid cancer. Contact your state authorities and inquire about what protections are in place in case of a nuclear reactor accident. For a complete list of specific sites per state, visit the Links Page on ThyCa's website (*www.thyca.org*).

TABLE 1.1

Nuclear Reactor States

A list of both commercial and government nuclear reactors, labs or

Alabama	Maine	North Carolina
Arizona	Maryland	Ohio
Arkansas	Massachusetts	Pennsylvania
California	Michigan	South Carolina
Connecticut	Minnesota	Tennessee
Florida	Mississippi	Texas
Georgia	Missouri	Vermont
Illinois	Nebraska	Virginia
Iowa	New Hampshire	Washington
Kansas	New Jersey	Wisconsin
Louisiana	New York	

nuclear facilities can be obtained from the United Nuclear Regulatory Commission as well as the International Nuclear Safety Center (INSC). Go to *www.thyca.org* for the online links.

2

FINDING (OR LOOKING FOR) LUMPS

This chapter may be a "day late and a dollar short" for many of you, who may be buying this book because you've just been diagnosed with thyroid cancer. (In that case, skip ahead to the chapter that discusses your cancer type.) But if you've bought this book because you're nervous about a lump in your neck, or think you may be at risk for thyroid cancer or a recurrence of your thyroid cancer, this is the chapter to read!

Thyroid Self Exam (TSE)

Every year, thousands of women find breast cancer lumps by doing Breast Self Exam (BSE). These types of self exams have been introduced as a tool to find early testicular cancers, skin cancers, and a host of others. This simple "lump finding" tool was introduced into the thyroid world in the mid-1990s. The Thyroid Self Exam is also known as the "Neck Check" and works along the same principles of BSE. The Neck Check was developed by the American Association of Clinical Endocrinologists. To do a neck check, you'll need a glass of water and a hand-held mirror. Here are the standard steps:

1. Hold the mirror in your hand, focusing on the area of your neck just below the Adam's apple (which some people confuse with the thyroid gland) and immediately above the collarbone.
2. While focusing on this area in the mirror, tip your head back slightly.
3. Take a drink of water and swallow. Normally, as you swallow, your windpipe raises and then goes back to its normal position.

4. As you swallow, look at your neck. Check for any bulges or a protrusion in this area when you swallow. (The thyroid gland is located further down on your neck, closer to the collarbone.) Repeat this a few times to be sure you're "all clear."

Over and above the standard TSE:

- Place your fingers at the back of your neck, at the top of your spine, and then knead your neck tissue towards the front like a piece of raw dough, feeling all the around to the front of your throat. Work the right side of your neck from back to front center, and then the left side from back to front center. You're looking for a painless lump anywhere from the size of a pea to the size of a golf ball.
- Feel all around the area just above the collarbone, or "pocket." (You're looking for the same thing.)

If you notice any bulges or lumps in these areas, see your doctor as soon as possible to have your lump investigated. If you have swollen lymph nodes in your neck or under your ears that persist for longer than one month, get them evaluated by a doctor. Your doctor can tell you if the lump is in the thyroid or not, possibly with the aid of ultrasound.

Investigating a Thyroid Lump/Nodule

Again, a lump is called a "nodule," which literally means "knot" and refers to a mass that can vary from the size of a pea to the size of a golf ball. Single thyroid nodules are usually one of three things: a growth that contains fluid (called a cyst); a growth that contains abnormal non-cancerous cells (called a benign tumor or adenoma); or a growth that contains cancerous abnormal cells (called a carcinoma). Cysts are frequently benign, and the majority of thyroid lumps are also benign.

Thyroid lumps are evaluated by the following types of doctors, listed in order of the least skilled in thyroid disease to the most skilled:

- Primary care doctors (family physicians, general practitioners, or internists).
- Endocrinologists (doctors specializing in the endocrine or hormone system).
- Thyroidologists (endocrinologists who only specialize in treating thyroid disease).

Fine Needle Aspiration Biopsy

A diagnostic procedure known as fine needle aspiration (FNA) has changed the way thyroid lumps are diagnosed. If you walked into your doctor's office with a lump on your neck 20 years ago, you'd have a thyroid scan (see further) and ultrasound, and you may have had the entire lump removed through a procedure known as excisional biopsy—a nasty little procedure that was used to diagnose my own thyroid cancer. You may have also been sent for an ultrasound to see if your lump was fluid-filled or solid or, with a scan, "hot" or "cold" – meaning that it's either sucking up iodine more than the other parts of the thyroid or relatively less. Well, these scans are rarely necessary today.

FNA, a 20-minute procedure, is basically considered the gold standard for evaluating a thyroid nodule. FNA is usually very accurate. It can be performed in a doctor's office, and is as simple as drawing a blood sample. The skin around your lump is cleansed with antiseptic before doing FNA. The needle (which is smaller than the standard needles used to sample blood), needs to be inserted three to six times to obtain a good sample. This is known as obtaining "passes," where each nodule is aspirated in different areas and in different directions. If you have several nodules, they'll each need to be aspirated with the appropriate number of passes with greater attention paid to larger nodules. FNA will suck out cells and/or fluid (fluid if it's a cyst), which is sent off to a pathologist (a specialist who examines cells), who is then able to determine if the lump is benign or malignant. FNA is usually very accurate. If your lump is a cyst, this procedure can also drain the cyst and collapse it, taking care of the problem entirely. FNA outweighs other diagnostic procedures in terms of the benefits; it's cheap, easy, fast, reasonably accurate and places far less stress on *you*, the patient. Studies show that because of FNA, cases of thyroid surgery have dropped by 50 percent. This means that many people can be spared "look-see surgery," which used to be done frequently when cancer was suspected. In some cases (such as when the lump can't be felt by the doctor), FNA is done using ultrasound to guide the needle.

Anytime you have FNA, it's a good idea to avoid medications that prolong blood clotting, such as aspirin. If you're on prescription medication, let your doctor know prior to the procedure. However, being on these medications doesn't mean you can't have this procedure done, it just reduces risks of bleeding. Once it's done, you'll have a bandage on the puncture site and then go home. You may have some neck tenderness or mild swelling afterwards, but you'll be fine in 24 hours. If you develop a fever, notice the puncture site becoming "black or blue" or begin bleeding, call your doctor. This may mean that you have a broken blood vessel or an infection at the puncture site.

FNA accuracy

Like many diagnostic procedures used to detect cancer, including Pap smears (which detect cervical cancer) and mammograms (breast imaging tests), FNA is not 100 percent accurate. Any physicians, including endocrinologists and internists, surgeons, pathologists, and radiologists, can perform FNAs if they're trained in the procedure. But FNA is not an exact science. Much depends on the skills of the doctor performing the FNA, his/her ability to obtain an adequate specimen of the right area, and the experience of the pathologist reading the slide that contains the smear. As a result, there are often "inconclusive" results, which occur about 10 to 15 percent of the time, or even "unsatisfactory," which occurs 1-10 percent of the time. A result that's inconclusive means that there's no way for the pathologist to tell whether the lump is benign or malignant. If you've been managed by a family doctor or internist up to this point, you may want to seek out an endocrinologist for a consultation. Sometimes the slides are sent to another pathologist who has more experience in interpreting thyroid cells (known as a "cytopathologist"). He or she can review the slides as well as interpret them. Otherwise, the rule is to either wait and repeat the FNA, or even go directly to surgery, depending upon the size and characteristics of the lump. An "unsatisfactory" FNA result means that the FNA procedure was not successful in obtaining enough thyroid cells for the pathologist to make a diagnosis (i.e., not enough "stuff" was obtained from the lump). In this case, the FNA may need to be performed by a more experienced doctor, or with the aid of ultrasound for guidance.

The tissue samples obtained through FNA have to be reviewed by a pathologist, a doctor who specializes in interpreting tissue samples. Pathologists who review cells specialize in cytology. Therefore, the results of an FNA are often dependent upon how much experience the pathologist has in cytology. In recent years, many reports about the shortage of pathologists, particularly in Canada, and their overwork, have surfaced. An overworked human pathologist is therefore capable of human error; when s/he's tired, s/he may make errors having to do with the interpretation of a sample. This can mean that cancerous tissue may be overlooked or not classified correctly. Or, tissue that's benign may be mistakenly labeled "cancerous," which can cause unnecessary stress, trauma and suffering. It is, therefore, resource shortages, rather than the FNA technology itself, which have created limitations to how accurate FNA can be. In smaller areas, many family doctors are not trained to do FNA, which also creates problems. Common pathology errors include:

- Calling tissue "malignant" (meaning cancerous) when it's benign (meaning, non-cancerous). This is called a false positive.
- Calling tissue "benign" when it's malignant. This is called a false negative.
- Identifying the malignant tumor correctly, but not classifying it as the right cell type or grade.
- Calling inadequate FNA samples "benign" because no cancer cells are seen. In order to be considered benign, the slides must contain sufficient numbers of non-cancerous thyroid cells.

A random study of pathology errors involving three major hospitals in the United States found that John Hopkins Hospital consistently had an error rate of 1.4 percent; a major hospital in Pennsylvania (Pennsylvania State Hershey Medical Center) had an error rate of 5.8 percent; while a major hospital in Massachusetts (University of Massachusetts Medical Center) had an error rate of 10.2 percent.

There are common problems, and then there are "errors." Common problems occur when there are simply not enough cells for the pathologist to sample to determine as much information as possible. And sometimes pathologists simply can't tell if the cells are malignant.

Confirming a pathology report

The only way to confirm a cancer diagnosis is through a biopsy of the tissue. If you receive news that your lump is (or might be) cancerous, you should get a second pathologist with more experience to review the biopsy slides and provide an independent, separate opinion. A qualified pathologist should be board certified in anatomic pathology and based in a university teaching hospital or major cancer center. At any one time, tissue samples are criss-crossing the country via Fedex for this very purpose!

If your doctor can't perform FNA...

Not all doctors are trained to do FNA. First, try to find someone with lots of experience who can perform it. Contact the Thyroid Cancer Survivors Association (Thyca) for a referral to a trained specialist in your area if you live in a remote or underserviced area. It's worth traveling the distance to find the right doctor to perform FNA.

Diagnostic Imaging Tests

An imaging test is used to evaluate lumps to determine a few things:

- Is the lump solid or fluid-filled?
- Does the rest of the thyroid gland look normal, or are there other lumps that can't be felt?
- Are these "hot" or "cold" nodules ("working" or "not working" nodules) on the thyroid (see further)?

For that, the best imaging test is a scan that involves a small dose of radioactive iodine, which normal thyroid cells absorb, and the imager picks up. Normal functioning thyroids will absorb radioactive iodine; these are known as "hot" nodules. Most benign and malignant nodules will not absorb radioactive iodine and are "cold" nodules. Also, most benign nodules are "cold" on scanning. A radioactive iodine scan involves taking pictures of your thyroid gland 24 hours after you ingest a small dose of radioactive iodine (called a tracer) or a simple tracer technetium, given by injection, which only requires a two-hour wait before imaging. Since most "hot" nodules occur in people with elevated thyroid hormone levels, scans should not be done if elevated levels are not present.

A "hot" nodule is a lump on the thyroid gland made up of functioning thyroid cells. Therefore, these lumps absorb the radioactive iodine eagerly. Chances are, if the nodule is functioning or "hot," it's not cancerous. In these cases, the lump found is either one of the nodules making up a multinodular goiter or is a solitary toxic adenoma (see further on).

A "cold" nodule, on the other hand, is made up of cells that have diminished ability to absorb iodine. However, only 10 percent of all cold nodules found turn out to be malignant. A cold nodule simply means that the cells making up the nodule are abnormal in that they absorb less iodine than the rest of the thyroid gland. But it's the nature of these cells that has yet to be determined—and that can only be done through an FNA biopsy. If your scan shows the presence of only hot nodules, your doctor will probably not bother to do a biopsy because cancerous cells are rarely hot. A cold nodule merely means that it's a suspicious nodule—not cancerous. Biopsies can help to determine whether a cold nodule is cancerous. For people with normal levels of thyroid hormone, only FNA biopsies, not scans, should be performed.

Ultrasound may be used to check structure, too, and can help to evaluate whether the lump was a cyst or solid. But today, ordering an ultrasound to evaluate thyroid nodules wouldn't typically give as much information as an FNA *unless* there was a questionable result with FNA, or a lump was difficult to see and biospy without the aid of an ultrasound.

Types of Lumps

Let's start with the good news: 85 percent of all thyroid lumps turn out to be benign. Lumps are often benign if you discover more than one of them, or if the rest of the thyroid gland itself is enlarged. Benign lumps also tend to be fleshier and softer, like the tip of your nose. Cancerous lumps tend to be hard, like the tip of your elbow. There are many kinds of benign lumps, which could be caused by inflammation of the thyroid (thyroiditis), discussed more in *The Thyroid Sourcebook*; secretions from the thyroid gland could also cause the lump (known as a colloid nodule). The following are other kinds of benign thyroid conditions or lumps:

- Multi-nodular goiter. The term multi-nodular means many nodules, as is the case with a multi-nodular goiter. What happens here is that normal functioning thyroid cells grow in places they don't belong, forming lumps outside the normal "boundaries" of where thyroid cells usually grow. The lumps can overproduce thyroid hormone, causing hyperthyroidism.
- Adenoma. This involves glandular cells, which usually clump together in a harmless, benign lump. Since the thyroid is a gland, any benign tumor that develops in the thyroid is called an adenoma. When abnormal cells grow in the thyroid gland, they vary in activity. Sometimes the cells are like "bumps on log;" they're lazy, inactive and are just "there" without a purpose. It's as though the cells develop and then lack the drive or capability to do anything else. They don't reproduce wildly, and they don't interfere with normal thyroid function; they simply exist. These cells live in a clump, and appear as a nodule in your thyroid. Since the FNA biopsy appearance of adenomas is similar to that of follicular cancers, most of these nodules require thyroid surgery to be properly classified.

- Solitary Toxic Adenoma. There can be another kind of benign growth, known as a solitary toxic adenoma. This is when the growth itself works overtime and produces too much thyroid hormone regardless of levels of thyroid stimulating hormone (see Introduction). The adenoma is "toxic" (not to be confused with malignant) in this case, because it causes hyperthyroidism. The adenoma hijacks the main function of the gland and assumes full production of thyroid hormone. The pituitary gland, which regulates thyroid stimulating hormone gets confused by the situation and turns off. What happens then is that there's no monitoring system in place and the adenoma makes too much thyroid hormone. A solitary toxic adenoma is a type of thyroid disorder and is not malignant. It's easily treated with radioactive iodine or anti-thyroid medications. For more information, see *The Thyroid Sourcebook*, 4th edition. Most of these nodules do not get biopsied because they produce "hot" nodules on thyroid scans.

Adenocarcinoma

About ten percent of the time, the lump will be diagnosed as an adenocarcinoma. The word *carcinoma* refers to a malignant growth that involves the epithelial cells. But when a tumor in a glandular area is malignant and stems from these epithelial cells, it's referred to as an adenocarcinoma. This often applies to thyroid cancer; although "adenocarcinoma" doesn't describe what kind of thyroid cancer you have. Chapters 3 through 5 discuss all the various types of thyroid cancer in detail, as well as the various treatments available for each type. Very rarely, the malignant tumor is not a thyroid tumor, but one that has spread from another organ, such as the lung, breast, or kidney. This book is limited, obviously, to a discussion of thyroid cancer.

Being diagnosed with any kind of cancer is like suddenly landing in a foreign country. You quickly realize language barriers, in the sense that everything is in MedicalSpeak; cultural barriers, in the sense that hospital life doesn't work like other environments you're used to; and a lack of comrades, in the sense that you suddenly feel isolated and are surrounded by strangers. So, cancer patients usually go through a crash course on their particular kind of cancer. They get educated, they learn how to navigate and maximize hospital visits, and they ultimately discover parts of themselves they never knew existed. The rest of this book operates like "landing gear." It will see you through the diagnosis, treatment and emotional journey of thyroid cancer.

3

All About Papillary and Follicular Cancers

The majority of thyroid cancers are either papillary or follicular, or sub-types of each. The words "papillary" and "follicular" refer to both the physical shape and personality of the cancer cells, as well as the behavior of the cells. In general, papillary is more likely to spread to lymph nodes in the neck and follicular is more aggressive with spread to distant sites, such as lung and bone. In other words, follicular is often a more danger-ous kind of cancer. This kind of cancer is extremely treatable and has an excellent survival rate. The "standard issue" thyroid cancer is papillary cancer. For women under 50 and men under 40, the cure rate is quite high. In the worst-case scenario, this cancer has a much smaller chance of recurrence, and a history of only less than five percent death rate. This is why many people think of it as "the good cancer."

Papillary Thyroid Cancer

Papillary tumors account for more than 75 percent of all thyroid cancers. The 10-year survival rate remains at 80 to 90 percent, meaning that 10 years after this diagnosis, 80 to 90 percent of people diagnosed with pap-illary thyroid cancer are still alive. If you have smaller papillary tumors, there's a 50 percent chance they've spread to the lymph nodes in the neck; if you have a larger papillary tumor, chances are about 75 percent that they've spread to the lymph nodes in the neck. The "pain in the neck" aspect of papillary thyroid cancer is that it tends to spread, creating a higher recurrence rate, but not a higher mortality rate. It's usually treatable. Most people with papillary cancer will not experience a spread beyond the neck. But sometimes there can be what's called a "distant metastasis" (metastasis means "spread") to the lung or bone. Papillary cancer tends to strike most often in people ages 30 through 50, and develops in women three times more frequently than men. The smaller the tumor, the better the news—as is the case with any cancer. Most thyroid cancers that are less than half an inch in size are considered to be the most treatable. Most thyroid cancers caused by radiation exposure are papillary cancers.

Tall Cell Papillary

Once you get papillary cancers under a microscope, things get a little more complicated because there are variations on types of papillary cancers. There are subtypes of thyroid cancer tumors—and some cell variants that can make the normally slow-growing papillary a little more aggressive. Having a "tall cell" variant of papillary thyroid cancer means you have a cancer that spreads more rapidly, and has a greater chance to lose the ability to suck up iodine. Because it spreads faster, recurrence is more likely, and you may require more vigilant follow-up than someone who has the usual papillary cancer. Meanwhile, more assertive surgery and follow-up care is required, considering the risk of spread.

Follicular Thyroid Cancer

Roughly ten percent of all thyroid cancers are purely follicular. This type of thyroid cancer tends to strike people over 40 more frequently than younger adults, and is not a type of thyroid cancer that commonly occurs as a direct result of radiation exposure. Age is the most important factor in figuring out how treatable follicular thyroid cancer is. If you are under 40, follicular thyroid cancer tends to be less aggressive than in people over 40; this is because it responds better to radioactive iodine therapy in younger people. Follicular thyroid cancer also tends to invade the veins and arteries of the thyroid gland, as well as distant organs, such as the lung, bone, brain, liver, bladder, and skin. Only about 15 percent of follicular cancers spread to the lymph nodes—a very different picture than what we see with papillary cancers. Purely follicular cancer is rare, and tends to strike most in people aged 40 to 60. Again, it strikes three times more often in women than men. As dismal as it sounds, the overall cure rate for purely follicular thyroid cancer is almost 95 percent in people under 40. After that, the cure rate depends greatly on the staging, discussed further on.

Hurthle Cell: a Close Relative

Hurthle cell thyroid cancer is a type of follicular thyroid cancer. When I was diagnosed with thyroid cancer in the early 1980s, no one even knew about the different clinical features of Hurthle cell cancer and it got "lumped in" (pardon the pun) with usual follicular cancer. This is an unusual type of tumor that's less common than follicular cancer, making up only 4 percent of all thyroid cancers. Under a microscope, a Hurthle cell is bigger than a usual follicular cell and turns dark pink when it's stained. Not sure if that helps you at all, but that's the difference under a microscope at the basic, cellular level! Most people who develop Hurthle cell thyroid cancer are in their mid-50s and beyond—about 10 years older than the follicular crowd. (Hurthle cell is reserved for the baby boomers.) Hurthle cell doesn't tend to spread to the lymph nodes, but can sprout again in the same place, or it can spread to the lung or bone. It takes years for Hurthle cell to grow and do much damage. The cure rate depends, like follicular, on the staging. Benign Hurthle cells can also be seen in many benign thyroid conditions, such as Hashimoto's disease and Graves' disease. (See *The Thyroid Sourcebook,* 4th edition for more on the latter.)

Not all Hurthle cell tumors are malignant, however. Some are benign adenomas, but it's usually not possible for a pathologist to determine whether this kind of tumor is benign or malignant with an FNA biopsy. You can only tell after you remove the thyroid gland and do a careful microscopic examination of the entire tumor. If you're lucky enough to find out if it's benign prior to any treatment after the first surgery, you do not require treatment because benign Hurthle cell tumors are not a threat to your health.

Staging and Spreading

Four people can be diagnosed with the same kind of thyroid cancer, but their treatments will depend on the stage of the cancer. To complicate matters, we also know that some cancers, such as tall cell papillary (see earlier), are more aggressive and may require more aggressive therapy. Most thyroid cancers have four stage classifications that basically answer the question "where has it spread?"

Papillary Stages

Stage I means that the cancer is confined to the thyroid in either one lobe or both lobes. Stage II in people under 45 means the cancer has spread beyond the thyroid; in people over 45, it means that the cancer may still be confined to the thyroid, but is larger than half an inch. If you're younger than 45, you won't get to Stage III; if you're older than 45, you might. This means the cancer has spread beyond the thyroid to surrounding lymph nodes, but has not gone beyond the neck. Stage IV is also only seen in people over 45, and means that the cancer has spread to distant organs, such as the lungs or the bones. Staging systems are not useful in predicting the outcomes of individual cases of thyroid cancer; they're mainly used as ways to predict general trends in thyroid cancer in large groups of patients.

Follicular Stages

Stage I means the cancer is confined to the thyroid, in either one lobe or both. Stage II in people under 45 means the cancer has spread beyond the thyroid gland. In people over 45, it means a larger tumor confined to the thyroid, of about half an inch in size. Stage III is seen only in people over 45, and means the cancer has spread outside the thyroid, possibly to the lymph nodes, but not beyond the neck. Stage IV, also seen only in people over 45, means the cancer has spread to distant organs, such as the lungs or bones.

Dealing with Diagnosis

When you're first told that you have a malignant lump, or are simply told you have "cancer," you'll be shocked. This can manifest into a variety of reactions from no reaction at all with some numbness to complete, high panic. In the latter, you may find your life flashing before your eyes, or you may not be able to think straight because your mind is racing in a hundred directions, and so on. Experts in the field of psycho-oncology, who specialize solely in dealing with patients' emotions and the many psychological issues of cancer diagnosis, classify the initial reaction of diagnosis into immobilization shock or high panic. Another phrase used is that of emotion vs. no emotion. Denial of the diagnosis is also a common reaction ("It can't be true; there's been a mistake" and so on), but denial often takes the form of denying the seriousness of the diagnosis or the urgency of the diagnosis (not to be confused with emergency).

What you must understand with any stage of papillary or follicular thyroid cancer is that this cancer diagnosis is *NOT* an emergency! You don't have to make the decisions regarding your treatment in the next 24 hours or even in the next week. It's taken a long time for your cancer to have reached the stage of discovery. As one specialist describes, diagnosis does not mean that your thyroid cancer has suddenly developed. It simply means that you now know something more about your body than you did a day ago.

I promise—two weeks in the life of a papillary or follicular thyroid cancer will not make any difference to your overall prognosis or survival. You're urged to take this time to absorb the information, educate yourself about your particular type of cancer (by perhaps buying a book like this one) and get a second opinion. In fact, many cancer centers today have a built-in second opinion structure, where a multidisciplinary team of specialists independently review each new diagnosis and, together, discuss their findings to make sure they all agree about the diagnosis, staging, and treatment recommendations.

Are You Sure?

If you're experiencing denial, which is a perfectly normal reaction to any cancer diagnosis, by all means use that denial to learn more. Here's what you can ask your specialist as well as any consulting specialist (i.e., the second opinion doctor) to make sure there's no mistake, which will help you deal with the information more comfortably. I've taken the liberty of wording the questions so that they can be used as a script (in case you're struggling for your own words). These would be appropriate questions to ask upon receiving the news that you have cancer, after a biopsy.

1. Are you basing this diagnosis solely on a single pathology report or have other specialists reviewed it? (Note: Although most of the time, the diagnosis of thyroid cancer is clear, doctors are generally cautioned never to accept a single pathology report as the last word, and to never tell patients they have cancer based on solely written or oral reports.)

2. Have you discussed my current health status and family history with other thyroid cancer specialists thoroughly so you can recommend an appropriate therapy for me, personally?

3. Has the pathologist reviewed enough samples to make an accurate diagnosis? (This is usually a "given" but it's helpful to have this information absolutely confirmed for your own level of comfort.)

4. Are you sure that the tissue samples the pathologist reviewed came from me? (Again, have this confirmed for your own level of comfort.)

5. Have you reviewed the pathology slides and report yourself? (This is key! Ask for a copy of the pathology report and ask your doctor to go over it with you and explain the report in language you can understand.)

6. Can I request a second look at my tissue samples from a separate institution? (If you're more comfortable...)

Your doctor or specialist should not be annoyed at your questions. At all. If s/he is, this is a bad sign and you should try to go elsewhere. In fact, most cancer specialists are more concerned about the patients who don't ask questions (they call this kind of person a "passive patient"). Unless you ask questions, your specialist has no way of knowing whether s/he's given you enough or appropriate information so that you can participate in treatment decisions.

Who Will Manage My Cancer Treatment?

Doctors work in teams to manage cancer therapy. This means that your primary care physician, surgeon (for thyroid surgery), endocrinologist (for thyroid hormone balancing), nuclear medicine specialist (for radioactive iodine treatment), radiation oncologist (in charge of external beam radiation therapy), and medical oncologist (in charge of chemotherapy for some advanced stages of thyroid cancer) are all involved with your treatment together. It's most common for the endocrinologist to act as the "project manager" for thyroid cancer management, coordinating the various treatments. Thyroid cancer surgeons can be head and neck surgeons, ear, nose and throat surgeons (called otolaryngologists), endocrine surgeons, or even general surgeons. The following questions will help you understand what's ahead:

1. Where can I go for more information? Ask to be referred to: a support group, a therapist, or a social worker who specializes in working with cancer patients.

2. Can you draw me a diagram of the cancerous parts of the thyroid, and shade in where the cancer is situated or has spread? Visualizing the cancer makes it easy to understand.

3. What stage is the cancer in?

4. Does your hospital or treatment center have a multidisciplinary cancer team? This means that a number of cancer specialists—pathologists, surgeons, radiation and medical oncologists—discuss your case together and recommend treatment options.

5. What treatment is being recommended and why? It's important to note that there are risks and benefits to certain treatment approaches. In order to make an informed choice, there are several things to be disclosed, discussed in the last section of this chapter.

6. Where and when will the treatments take place, and how long will they last? This will help you in short- and long-term planning. For example, if you're having radioactive iodine therapy (see chapter 6), you'll need to be in isolation for a period of time.

7. What other health problems should I be on the look out for during treatment? Ask about all the side effects for each treatment recommended, which can include numbness in the neck from cut nerves, dry mouth from radioactive iodine therapy, and problems surrounding calcium as a result of "nicks" to your parathyroid glands (see further). Voice changes and salivary gland abnormalities can also occur.

8. How can I contact my managing doctor between visits?

9. Can I take other medications during treatments? Or, how will the treatments affect other medications I'm taking? It's a good idea to carry a card listing all other prescription and non-prescription medications you're taking. You may also want to list any herbal therapies on this card, too.

10. What about alcohol? Considering what you're going through, you might want a glass of wine or a shot of hard liquor occasionally.

Telling a Life Partner or Spouse

Thyroid cancer affects your entire family. It's important to keep in mind that your spouse will be going through as much fear and shock as you. But in some ways, there may be an even greater feeling of helplessness because there's nothing s/he can do to make it better or make it go away. But communication breakdown usually develops if you hide your own feelings for fear that they'll frighten your spouse. So try not to do this; try to be honest about your feelings, because this helps to include your spouse in the process. Telling your spouse what s/he can do for you will make him or her feel as though s/he's capable, even in a small way, of lessening the burden of the diagnosis. At the same time, it's important to share what you're going through whenever you need to talk. Indeed, you may find that initially the atmosphere in the home may change hourly, revolving around you ("Are you okay?" "Do you want to talk now?"). Go with the flow and try not to be angry with a continuous checking in. This is your family's way of caring and you need to let yourself be cared for. In fact, giving yourself permission is perhaps the hardest thing to do after a cancer diagnosis. Permission to feel bad; permission to feel needy; permission to let others care for you.

Of course, there are some exceptions to the rule. Some spouses may not have the coping skills necessary to deal with the situation and may even get angry about the diagnosis or leave the house to work it out. Obviously, this is a sign that there are fundamental problems in your relationship anyway; the diagnosis is not causing this behavior, it's simply bringing the truth about the relationship to the surface faster. In these cases, family therapy, counseling and spousal cancer support groups (support groups for the spouses of cancer patients) are important steps to take so you can resolve your feelings about the diagnosis in a healthy way. Chapter 8 covers psychosocial support issues in much more detail.

Telling Small Children

Small children are intuitive beings who will sense something's wrong in the home. In fact, hiding the diagnosis from a small child is the worst thing you can do. Hiding a diagnosis may lead the child to conclude that s/he is the cause of your illness, for example. Cancer therapists recommend explaining the situation to a child in language s/he can understand, and if necessary, explaining or retelling it over and over again. The tendency is for younger children to repeatedly ask the same questions. This is their way of finding bearings in a new situation. Hearing the same response helps to build consistency into a new reality.

The well partner or spouse should continue his/her routine with the children and watch for behavior changes. For example, young children may suddenly have difficulty at school, difficulty sleeping, increased upset and tantrum-like scenes, separation anxiety from the well or ill parent, as well as unusual creative expression of the situation, such as disturbing arts and crafts. A classic example of the latter is the child who suddenly draws pictures of monsters eating or attacking his/her ill parent.

Again, no matter how well you explain your illness or how open you are with your child, exceptions apply, and some children will have more difficulty adjusting. You should seek out family and child counseling if you're worried about a child's behavior. For more information about dealing with radioactive iodine (RAI) therapy and small children, see chapter 6.

Your Treatment Options

I want to stress that you *do* have options with respect to thyroid cancer treatment; I never knew I did when I was treated, however. The options revolve around your current health status, quality of life, and your comfort level surrounding conservative treatment approaches or more aggressive treatment approaches. Regardless of which stage your papillary or follicular cancer is in, you always have options, and the right to informed consent (see further on). Treating thyroid cancer always involves surgery, but there are different kinds of surgeries. For example, a partial thyroidectomy removes only half the thyroid gland. A total thyroidectomy removes the entire thyroid gland. A neck dissection removes lymph nodes in the neck that contain cancer.

Beyond surgery, there are options of further treatment, which include:

- Radioactive iodine (RAI) therapy. This depends on the stage of your cancer, and whether you have a more aggressive form of cancer (such as follicular or tall cell papillary). This involves taking a capsule or liquid form of RAI. Because the thyroid absorbs iodine, any differentiated thyroid cancer cells, such as papillary and follicular, should absorb the radioactive iodine, too, which will kill them. You have the option to refuse this procedure or to be fully informed prior to consent.

- External beam radiation therapy. Generally reserved for a more advanced stage, or aggressive types of thyroid cancer, which do not take up radioactive iodine, this involves using high-dose X-rays or other similar high-energy rays to kill cancer cells. This is an option that probably won't be presented unless your thyroid cancer progresses in spite of surgery and RAI. You have the option to refuse this treatment or to be fully informed prior to consent.

- Hormone therapy. When your thyroid gland is removed, you will be hypothyroid, which I discuss thoroughly in my book, *The Hypothyroid Sourcebook*, as well as further on in this book. So you'll need to be on replacement thyroid hormone, known as levothyroxine sodium (T4), in order to function at all. This generally doesn't happen right away, however, because it takes a week for half of the thyroid hormone in your body to be used up (that is, the "half-life" is a week). You'll need to be off any thyroid hormone after surgery in order for the thyroid stimulating hormone (TSH) to rise high enough to do a whole body scan to detect whether there are any thyroid cancer cells left. That is what determines the next wave of treatments. But once you're clear of cancer, you'll also require a "suppression dosage" to keep your TSH level very low in order to prevent it from "waking up" surviving thyroid cancer cells that may have persisted at microscopic levels after your treatment. As one endocrinologist put it, TSH is a "fertilizer" for thyroid cancer cells, which is why you need to keep it suppressed. You have options in this case regarding: (1) your medication brand, and whether you need to add another medicine to prevent any rapid heart beats from the slightly higher than normal T4 dose (this may be a type of beta-blocker, which slows down the heart rate); and (2) whether you want to go off your medication for follow-up scans (see chapter 7). If you refuse to take thyroid hormone replacement at all, you won't function for very long and your life will be in jeopardy. In addition, there's a controversy regarding whether adding T3 (Cytomel®) to T4 treatment has any benefits. But you may want to be informed about complementary therapies that can improve your health and well being during bouts of hypothyroidism or to aid with the absorption of thyroid hormone. Complementary therapy is discussed in chapter 9. For those of you who have a papillary cancer that's less than one cm in size at a single site within the thyroid gland, and the tumor has not invaded blood vessels or lymph nodes, you may not require scans or a TSH suppression dosage.

Recommendations by Stage

The exact stage of your thyroid cancer is not the only type of information that directly determines the type of treatment you should receive. Nonetheless, since some sources use it in their approach, here is a general idea of how it may affect your treatment.

For stage I papillary, and stage I follicular, the treatment involves removing some (for single papillary cancers less than one cm in size) or all of the thyroid gland (for all the rest). (See next section on partial vs. total thyroidectomy.) Thyroid hormone replacement therapy on a TSH-suppression dosage is the next step, which is usually preceded by RAI therapy.

For stage II papillary and stage II follicular, the treatment is the same, except the entire thyroid gland will be removed, and a neck dissection will be done (removing the lymph nodes that contain cancer).

For stage III papillary and stage III follicular, the treatment is the same as above, except there may be higher RAI doses and more frequent evaluations.

For stage IV papillary and follicular (after a total thyroidectomy and neck dissection, as well as thyroid hormone therapy), you may have many of the following: very high dose RAI, external beam radiation for tumors which do not respond to RAI, and perhaps further surgeries to remove recurrent tumor or tumors which have spread to dangerous locations (for example: spine, brain, bones).

For Hurthle cell tumors, the whole thyroid is always removed because Hurthle cell can be more aggressive. It is important to take sufficient RAI therapy after surgery to get the best chance to destroy these cancer cells since at least one third of the time these tumor cells lose the ability to suck up the RAI. Additional tests and close follow-up is necessary to safeguard against this possibility.

General Treatment Plans

Papillary thyroid cancers that are one cm or less in size (less than half an inch), exist as a single tumor within the thyroid gland, and show no evidence of any spread to the neck or elsewhere, can be treated with surgery alone (usually removal of half of the thyroid; a lobectomy). These small papillary cancers do not require radioactive iodine scans or treatments. Many physicians will have you take sufficient T4 to keep the TSH slightly less than normal, although some people may not be told to take any T4 at all.

All other papillary cancers and all follicular thyroid cancers of any size require a total (or near total) removal of the thyroid and removal of any lymph nodes in the neck likely to contain tumor. This is followed by radioactive iodine (RAI) therapy, followed by nuclear medicine tests using small RAI doses to search for the recurrence of tumors with whole body scanning. Usually, by six months after the first RAI treatment, a whole body scan and thyroglobulin assessment is made (see chapter 7) to make sure that all evidence of thyroid cancer is gone. If so, then these assessments are repeated with longer and longer intervals between them. If not, then the RAI treatment is repeated (no closer than five to six months apart) until all the tests show you to be free of tumor

For medullary thyroid cancers, and for those papillary and follicular cancers that are persistent and unresponsive to RAI, there are no definitive treatments aside from surgery. In some situations, external beam radiotherapy can be used; however tumors that have spread beyond the neck are rarely treatable with current methods. Anaplastic thyroid cancers are both rare and extremely dangerous, requiring immediate involvement of specialist physicians from the earliest moment that they are discovered. (Your doctor can telephone these specialists for a consultation.)

Partial vs. Total Thyroidectomy

There are a few different kinds of thyroid surgery. The majority of thyroid cancer patients will have a total thyroidectomy and modified neck dissection. This involves removing all of the thyroid gland and nearby lymph nodes that are cancerous. Partial thyroidectomy is reserved for people with small papillary cancers (under one cm in diameter), and can involve a few types of procedures. One procedure involves removing one lobe (lobectomy). Another procedure, called a "lobectomy and isthmusectomy", involves removing one lobe and the isthmus, which is bridge of tissue linking the lobes together (like the horizontal line in an H). There's also something called a near-total thyroidectomy or subtotal thyroidectomy, which removes the tumor from the cancerous side of the gland, as well as the isthmus and most of the other lobe. As long as the piece of thyroid gland that's been left behind is minimal (less than 2 gm by weight), it can be considered, essentially, a total thyroidectomy. There's absolutely no reason for any surgeon to purposely remove only part of a thyroid lobe or to remove the cancerous nodule by itself, unless the tumor is so aggressively invading into the neck that he or she cannot do more surgery safely. For the purpose of this book, I'll define anything that's not a total thyroidectomy as a "partial thyroidectomy."

Total thyroidectomy vs. partial thyroidectomy is an extremely controversial issue right now with thyroid surgeons and endocrinologists. Some surgeons may want to leave as much thyroid tissue intact as possible. This partial thyroidectomy is only acceptable if you have a single papillary cancer nodule less than one cm in size with no evidence of spread to any other area. This is because such small papillary cancers will rarely cause further problems for you after such surgery. Otherwise, the only appropriate choice should be between a "total" thyroidectomy and a "near-total" thyroidectomy. This is because these cancers have a reasonably high chance of having spread to the opposite side of the thyroid gland and beyond the thyroid gland, into the neck or more distant sites. Very experienced "thyroid" surgeons who perform many thyroid surgeries each year (more than 25 cases) feel capable of doing "total" thyroidectomies, while surgeons with fewer cases or less experience often want to leave small pieces of the thyroid gland behind (usually near the vocal cord nerves or parathyroid glands), a "near total" thyroidectomy.

The vocal cord nerves (the recurrent laryngeal nerves) on each side pass near (or into) the thyroid gland. If one nerve is damaged, then the vocal cord it connects to becomes paralyzed, causing a hoarse or weak voice. If both nerves become damaged then there may be a need for a hole to be made in the windpipe (a tracheostomy) to permit you to breathe. Sometimes the tumor itself causes this problem by eating its way into these nerves. The most experienced surgeons are least likely to cause such problems; however these are known risks of this surgery and should be carefully explained to you before you consent to the surgery. It's good practice to ask the surgeon about the frequency with which these problems have occurred in his or her other patients and about his or her own experience and training in this surgery.

Another complication that's even more frequent is caused by damage to the parathyroid glands. These four tiny glands are found near the thyroid gland and can be mistaken by the surgeon for lymph nodes. They make parathyroid hormone (PTH), which tells the body how to manage its calcium level. PTH makes the kidneys hold on to calcium from the blood, and activates Vitamin D to make it more effective in absorbing calcium from the intestines. The loss of PTH makes calcium leak out in the urine and keeps it from being replenished from the diet. Low calcium levels resulting from damage to all four parathyroid glands cause numbness, tingling sensations around the lips, mouth, hands and feet, muscle cramps, twitching, and sometimes even seizures. (I've provided an excerpt from a thyroid cancer survivor's story of hypoparathyroidism at the end of this chapter.) Most often, these glands are "bruised" during the surgery and the low calcium levels only last a couple of days. Sometimes they are permanently lost and daily treatment with activated forms of high-dose Vitamin D and large daily doses of calcium supplements are needed forever.

Despite these potential problems, it may be worth having a "total" thyroidectomy to absolutely minimize your risk of recurrence and prevent the scenario of a repeat thyroid surgery (I know people who've been through this too, and it's not fun!). Repeat thyroid surgery also involves working through previous scar tissue, which can take longer and may involve more complications. Having another surgery performed in the same site as a previous thyroid surgery makes having problems with damaged parathyroid glands and paralyzed vocal cords far more likely. This is why you'd never want a surgeon to remove part of a thyroid lobe, putting you at risk for another surgery on that same side.

In "total" thyroidectomy surgery with very experienced thyroid surgeons, there's roughly a two percent chance of permanent damage to the nerves of the voice box or parathyroid glands. But considering that only two percent of the population gets thyroid cancer at all, "two percent" is not such a low percentage to us thyroid cancer patients. You'll have to weigh that two percent risk against the fact that thyroid cancer patients with total thyroidectomy (followed by radioiodine therapy and thyroid suppression) have a significantly lower recurrence rate of their cancers (when their papillary tumors are greater than one cm). Also, the less normal thyroid tissue left in your body, the greater the benefit of RAI therapy after surgery. This is because RAI therapy following a thyroidectomy is an important way to eradicate the thyroid cells that are frequently left behind—all potentially cancerous tissue! It's also an important way to detect a recurrence of thyroid cancer. But if there's half a thyroid gland still left inside you, radioactive iodine therapy isn't all that effective because it will probably wind up in the intact lobe left behind, causing thyroiditis (this happens about 60 percent of the time). And a radioactive iodine scan is useless because it's designed to pick up thyroid remnants that can't be seen with the naked eye. The bottom line is that the more thyroid tissue left inside you, the more potential there is for it to become cancerous and, therefore, for you to have to repeat all the diagnostic tests as well as surgery.

The second surgeon consult

When it comes to the diagnosis of thyroid cancer, getting a second opinion means that you see two separate doctors about the same biopsy report to see if the diagnoses match. But when it comes to thyroid surgery and treatment options, you might also see two separate doctors about treatment recommendations to see if the *recommendations* match. In general, if a partial thyroidectomy is recommended, it's wise to consult another surgeon before consenting. Or, if a total thyroidectomy is recommended for a small stage I papillary tumor, it's also wise to consult a second surgeon. Often, a follicular cancer can't be distinguished from a benign follicular adenoma until the pathologist has had several days to examine the slides from the first partial thyroidectomy. If a cancer is found, the surgeon will need to do a second surgery to remove the other thyroid lobe. Some cancers, such as medullary thyroid cancer and anaplastic thyroid cancer, require more detailed and aggressive surgery, which may be beyond the expertise of the first surgeon. Finally, anyone diagnosed with tall cell papillary would be wise to consult a surgeon regarding the post-surgery options. (In this case a "total" thyroidectomy would likely be recommended by all knowledgeable surgeons).

Questions to ask before surgery

1. Should I be concerned about drug interactions? If you're taking any prescription drug whatsoever, make sure you disclose the name of the drug and find out how long before the surgery you need to be off of that drug. A class of drugs known as non-steroidal anti-inflammatories (NSAIDs) can be particularly dangerous. The same goes for any over-the-counter drug, be it ibuprofen, acetaminophen, or aspirin. Some people may be on blood-thinning medication and require special preparation for surgery.

2. What's the likelihood of my needing a blood transfusion? If there's a good chance of this, you may wish to consider what's called *autologous transfusion*. This may reduce the chance of infection with a blood-borne virus from a transfusion, as well as the demand on the public blood supply. There is now a drug called Procrit, which is recombinant human erythropoietin that's used to reduce the need for a blood transfusion. This is a drug that is identical to your body's erythropoietin (the hormone that stimulates the manufacture of red blood cells), and increases your red blood cell count prior to surgery.

3. How long do I need to fast prior to surgery? Also find out what foods you should stay away from before and after the procedure, and so on. Usually you'll be told to have your last solids 6 hours prior to surgery and your last liquids 3 hours prior to surgery. You should also make sure that your surgeon avoids evaluating you with CAT scans that use iodine-containing contrast dyes since they can interfere with your RAI therapy after surgery for many months.

Informed Consent and Thyroid Cancer

You need to have full information in order to make the necessary decisions about your treatment. You should be aware that you're not just entitled to information, but legally owed information. Being informed about medical tests and procedures is known as "informed consent," which is a guiding ethical principle for medical practitioners and researchers. It means that in order for someone to make an informed decision, there must be full disclosure of all risks and benefits; that person must completely understand what's being explained; that person must be fully competent; and that person must feel free to say "yes" or "no" according to his/her own wishes, values, and "gut feelings" without any coercion or coaxing.

Most medical ethicists agree that informed consent is an oxymoron, like "jumbo shrimp"—the two ideas are incompatible. Because to be truly informed when it comes to many medical procedures (thyroid or otherwise), it's often not good enough to know "what time it is;" you need to know how to build a watch. The problem with "informed consent" is that unless *you* are a doctor, too, how informed can you really become?

So, whenever you consent to any kind of medical test, procedure or treatment, here are all the things your doctor should be disclosing:

- A description of the test, procedure, or treatment and its expected effects (e.g., duration of hospital stay, expected time to recovery, restrictions on daily activities, scars);
- Information about relevant alternative options and their expected benefits and relevant risks; and
- An explanation of the consequences of declining or delaying treatment.

Your doctor should also be giving you an opportunity to ask questions—and should be available to answer them. However, there are also some questions you should ask yourself:

- Do *you* understand the information relevant to your decision and do you appreciate the reasonably foreseeable consequences of your decision or *lack* of decision? This is what's known as your *capacity* to consent to procedures. If you're upset or your head is spinning from too much technical jargon being hurled at you all at once, you may not have the capacity to truly consent.
- Do you understand what's being disclosed and can you make your decision based on this information?
- Are you being allowed to make your decision free of any undue influences? (For example, are you in pain? Is information being distorted or omitted? Are you being sedated?) This is what's known as *voluntariness*; involuntary consent means, of course, that you haven't consented to a procedure.

If you answer "no" to any of these questions, you are probably not being given adequate information, or you are in no shape to make a decision about your health. In this case, you may want to book a separate "Q and A" session with your doctor to make sure you can give your informed consent.

What to Expect after Surgery

If you talk to thyroid cancer survivors, most of them barely remember the surgery; it's what happens after that's the biggest pain in the neck—going through life without a thyroid gland. You'll become hypothyroid, which means "low or no thyroid hormone" in your body (see next section) unless you take your thyroid hormone medication.

More immediate post-surgery concerns might be around scar care, however. The scar thyroidectomy procedures leave is sometimes called a "necklace scar," because the incision mimics the line of a thin necklace. Plastic surgery techniques are used to minimize the scar. My scar is barbaric compared to what I see today; but even in my case, my scar is not disfiguring and barely noticeable (even though, because of neck dissection, it travels up the right side of my neck behind my ear). The right necklace completely covers it. Standard scar lengths measure roughly four to five inches in length, but scars can be as small as three inches. These incisions, without any skin care typically heal very well. But pure vitamin E oil, and the essential oils of rose, frankincense, helichrysum, and hyssop are all known for healing scar tissue. You can also blend these oils together, using pure vitamin E oil as a base. Some people (especially those with darker skin) can form keloids. If this is the case, discuss this with your surgeon ahead of time. Also consult chapter 9 on complementary medicine.

Numbness and Nerve Damage

Thyroid surgery frequently involves cutting nerve endings in the neck area, which can leave parts of your neck and shoulder area numb. It can take years for these nerve endings to grow back. Some thyroid cancer survivors have had numbness around ear lobes and even the tongue. In my own case, after more than 20 years post-surgery, I still have no feeling on the right side of my neck and shoulder below it. If I scratch my ear lobe on the right side, I feel it in my neck—the result of confused signals from the nerve endings growing back. Each of you will have different types of numbness that can often be helped through massage or acupuncture (see chapter 9). Sometimes you can still feel itches on the numb regions, but lack the ability to scratch. This can be maddening, but is controlled through creams recommended by a dermatologist.

Hypothyroidism

Being hypothyroid means that your thyroid gland is not making enough (or in this case, any) thyroid hormone for your body's requirements. When you're hypothyroid, everything slows down— including your body temperature. The most common hypothyroid symptoms include:

- *Cardiovascular changes.* An unusually slow pulse (between 50 and 70 beats per minute), and either too low or too high blood pressure. Higher cholesterol and fluid retention may occur, too.
- *Cold intolerance.* You may not be able to find a comfortable temperature, and may often wonder "why it's always so *freezing* in here?!" This is because your entire metabolic rate has slowed down as your body conserves heat by diverting blood away from your skin.
- *Depression.* You may find that your mood "flatlines" and you exhibit symptoms of major depression, including empty mood, loss of interest in formerly pleasureable activities, and loss of appetite (which you won't notice due to weight gain for other reasons). See my book, *50 Ways To Fight Depression Without Drugs* or *Women and Depression* for more on depression.

- *Digestive changes and weight gain.* Because your system is slowed down, you'll suffer from constipation, hardening of the stools and bloating (which may cause bad breath), and poor appetite, as well as heartburn.
- *Fatigue and sleepiness.* The most classic symptom is a distinct, lethargic tiredness or sluggishness, causing you to feel unnaturally sleepy. I refer to my own hypothyroid symptoms as "ass draggy." Researchers now know that when you're hypothyroid, you're unable to reach the deepest "stage 4" level of sleep, which is the most restful kind of sleep. This is why you'll remain tired, sleepy, and unrefreshed.
- *Menstrual cycle changes.* Menstrual periods can become much heavier and more frequent than usual, and sometimes ovaries can stop producing an egg each month. This can make conception difficult, if you're trying to have a child. For more details, see *The Thyroid Sourcebook for Women.* If you're suffering from more severe PMS, consult my book *Managing PMS Naturally.*
- *Muscular aches.* Common complaints from hypothyroid people are muscular aches and cramps (which may contribute to crampier periods).
- *Poor memory and concentration.* Hypothyroidism causes a "spacey" feeling, where you may find it difficult to remember things, or to concentrate at work.
- *Skin changes.* Skin may feel dry and coarse to the point where it flakes like powder when you scratch it. Cracked skin will also become the norm on your elbows and kneecaps.
- *Hoarseness.* You may find that you're speaking in a hoarse, monotonous voice.

Most thyroid cancer patients will receive thyroid hormone after surgery until they require a whole body scan (see chapter 7). Generally, thyroid replacement hormone will rebalance your thyroid hormone level in your body, and you'll begin to feel more like yourself. Thyroid medication is also discussed in chapter 7. To check for hypothyroidism, a TSH test is done. A normal TSH reading ranges from 0.5 to 5. A reading greater than 5 suggests that you're hypothyroid, while a reading less than 5 suggests that you're hyperthyroid (meaning that you're on too high a dose of thyroid hormone). It's important to remember that most people with thyroid cancer are purposely given sufficient thyroid hormone to keep the TSH under 0.1 and are just a tiny bit hyperthyroid in a safe fashion.

Hypothyroidism is a complex topic. For more information, please consult *The Hypothyroid Sourcebook*, which not only explains hypothyroid symptoms in more detail, but provides a proactive program I have designed to help you manage hypothyroidism. In it you'll find The Hypothyroid Diet, The Hypothyroid Active Living Program, and The Hypothyroid Herbal and Wellness Program.

Songs about Hypo Symptoms

Megan Stendebach, a thyroid cancer survivor (she was diagnosed in 1997), is the "Weird Al" of the thyroid world. Using humor to educate people about hypothyroid symptoms, she has created a funny and warm website you can go to (*www.thyroidcancersongs.com*). Reproduced with permission here are three of her tunes.

My God, I'm A Hypo Boy!

Remember how John Denver made the world seem so simple? Join me now in singing this perky song, "My God, I'm A Hypo Boy!"

Well life on the couch is kinda laid back
Ain't much an old hypo boy like me can't hack
It's late to rise and early in the sack
My God, I'm a hypo boy!

Well a sluggish kinda life never did me no harm
Dozin' on my family and missin' the alarm
My days are all filled with a lazy hypo charm
My God, I'm a hypo boy!

When my nap's all done and sun's settin' low
I pull out my bathrobe and I tie it kinda low
Can't see me feet but they're somewhere down below
My God, I'm a hypo boy!

I'd rather be snorin' all day if I could
But the boss and my wife wouldn't take it very good
So I sleep when I can, work when I should
My God, I'm a hypo boy!

(Chorus)
Well I got me some Synthroid, maybe too little
When the sun's comin' up I got flab on my middle
Life ain't nothin' but a pesky hypo riddle
My God, I'm a hypo boy!

Well I would trade my life for diamonds or jewels
I've always been one of those hyper-hungry fools
I'd rather have a middle so my wife kinda drools
My God, I'm a hypo boy!

Hyper folks have energy and stay pretty lean
A lotta hypo people think that's mighty keen
Well folks let me tell ya now exactly what I mean
My God! I'm a hypo boy!

(Chorus)
Well I got me some Synthroid, maybe too little
When the sun's comin' up I got flab on my middle
Life ain't nothin' but a pesky hypo riddle
My God, I'm a hypo boy!

Well, they'll fiddle with my dosage til the day I die
Doin' what they can to get my TSH right
Sometimes it's low, sometimes it's high
My God, I'm a hypo boy!

My endo told me, "Son, your dosage is a riddle
Ya oughta feel fine, just as fit as a fiddle.
But you feel like a slug, so we'll raise it just a little."
My God, I'm a hypo boy!

(Chorus)
Well I got me some Synthroid, maybe too little
When the sun's comin' up I got flab on my middle
Life ain't nothin' but a pesky hypo riddle
My God, I'm a hypo boy!

Oh, My Rear, My Big Fat Rear

Imagine Julie Andrews and the Von Trapp Family Singers going hypothyroid...

Oh:	my rear, my big fat rear
Hey:	this hypo isn't fun
Me:	a shame - I'm not myself
Fog:	my brain - it cannot run
So:	I think I'll go to bed
Blah:	to bloat and wallow so
Tea:	something to warm my head

That will bring us back to HYpo, HYpo!

(Sing it again!)

The Twelve Weeks of Hypo Hell

OK, kids! It's time for a Sing-Along! This one goes out to all you Hypo-ites out there. Sing it to the tune of "The Twelve Days of Christmas. A-one and a-two....

In the first week of hypo hell
my symptoms gave to me
the need for a really great nap.

In the second week of hypo hell
my symptoms gave to me
two migraine headaches,
and the need for a really great nap.

In the third week of hypo hell
my symptoms gave to me
three seafood cravings,
two migraine headaches,
and the need for a really great nap.

In the fourth week of hypo hell
my symptoms gave to me
four bouts of weeping,
three seafood cravings,
two migraine headaches,
and the need for a really great nap.

In the fifth week of hypo hell
my symptoms gave to me
FIVE SLEEPLESS NIGHTS!
Four bouts of weeping,
three seafood cravings,
two migraine headaches,
and the need for a really great nap.

In the sixth week of hypo hell
my symptoms gave to me
six pounds of weight gain,
FIVE SLEEPLESS NIGHTS!

Four bouts of weeping,
three seafood cravings,
two migraine headaches,
and the need for a really great nap.

In the seventh week of hypo hell
my symptoms gave to me
seven days of dry skin,
six pounds of weight gain,
FIVE SLEEPLESS NIGHTS!
Four bouts of weeping,
three seafood cravings,
two migraine headaches,
and the need for a really great nap.

In the eighth week of hypo hell
my symptoms gave to me
eight constipations,
seven days of dry skin,
six pounds of weight gain,
FIVE SLEEPLESS NIGHTS!
Four bouts of weeping,
three seafood cravings,
two migraine headaches,
and the need for a really great nap.

In the ninth week of hypo hell
my symptoms gave to me
nine aching muscles,
eight constipations,
seven days of dry skin,
six pounds of weight gain,
FIVE SLEEPLESS NIGHTS!
Four bouts of weeping,
three seafood cravings,
two migraine headaches,
and the need for a really great nap.

In the tenth week of hypo hell
my symptoms gave to me
ten frozen fingers,
nine aching muscles,
eight constipations,
seven days of dry skin,
six pounds of weight gain,
FIVE SLEEPLESS NIGHTS!
Four bouts of weeping,
three seafood cravings,
two migraine headaches,
and the need for a really great nap.

In the eleventh week of hypo hell
my symptoms gave to me
eleven memory lapses,
and I forget the rest...

In the twelfth week of hypo hell
my symptoms gave to me
twelve temper tantrums,
eleven memory lapses,
ten frozen fingers,
nine aching muscles,
eight constipations,
seven days of dry skin,
six pounds of weight gain,
FIVE SLEEPLESS NIGHTS!
Four bouts of weeping,
three seafood cravings,
two migraine headaches,
and THE NEED FOR A REALLY GREAT NAP!!!

Treatments After Surgery

Most thyroid cancer patients will become intimately acquainted with radioactive iodine, which is used for both scanning and treatment. This is complicated stuff, and for that reason, I have dedicated chapter 6 to the topic. Follow-up scans, and sometimes recurrence of thyroid cancer are the norm. There may also be cases where external beam radiation is recommended. This is all discussed in chapter 7. Chemotherapy is rarely involved in the treatment of thyroid cancer. It is reserved for anaplastic cancer, where new and effective chemotherapy is needed for this terribly aggressive tumor. See chapter 5 for more details on chemotherapy.

Hypoparathyroidism

Everyone has at least four parathyroid glands that control the blood calcium level, or calcium balance (some people have more than four!). These glands are located on the back of each lobe of your thyroid gland. The easiest way to get a handle on their exact location is to imagine the capital letter H. At each tip of the H, imagine a circle. If the H is your thyroid gland, the circles at each tip are your parathyroid glands.

Because the glands are so close in proximity to the thyroid gland, a surgeon must be careful not to touch or disrupt the parathyroid glands. As long as there's one good functioning parathyroid gland, there's no problem. However, these small glands are susceptible to either temporary or permanent damage during thyroid surgery.

If the parathyroid glands were to become accidentally removed or damaged from thyroid surgery, your blood calcium levels would drop (known as hypocalcemia) and your blood phosphorous levels would increase (known as hyperphosphatemia). This occurs because of inadequate parathyroid hormone (PTH) production. Symptoms can range from quite mild tingling in the hands, fingers, and around the mouth to more severe forms of muscle cramps. Surgeons will tell you it almost *never* happens. But this makes people who experience it feel diminished and quite isolated. The unfortunate reality is that some people will have to live with this problem. For this reason, I have provided, with permission, a personal story of hypoparathyroidism, sent to me by one of the founding members of the Canadian Thyroid Cancer Support Group (Thry'vors).

Doctors quote really low levels of permanent hypoparathyroidism (HPTH), but hearing some real life stories made me nervous. If it's so rare, then what are the odds that I would work with someone who not only has it, but has also met others with the same thing? I questioned who to believe more—doctors or patients, and I became frustrated because no one really knows. I've concluded that the parathyroids must be one of the least understood glands in the entire body.

I had a total thyroidectomy in September of 2000, at the age of 32. I spent a lot of time worrying about what the scar was going to look like, how to hide it, and whether I could handle having temporary or permanent HPTH, the symptoms of which range from tingling and numbness in the extremities (lips, hands, and feet) to seizures. I accepted that a lot of patients have temporary problems, but permanent problems? When and how do you know it's permanent? How bad is this going to be?

I could tell my calcium level had dropped (hypocalcemia) while in recovery, because of the tingling in my hand. My surgeon and his residents reported seeing two parathyroid glands during the surgery and that neither had turned gray, something that parathyroid glands often do. None of my parathyroid glands were removed (later confirmed by the pathology report), so it is really unexplainable why my calcium level dropped so low. While in the hospital, I had intravenous calcium, but also started taking calcium supplements with a drug called Rocaltrol® (calcitriol).

Rocaltrol (synthetic calcitriol) is a vitamin D metabolite that helps absorb calcium. It's the most activated known form of vitamin D. Normally the vitamin D3 that the body produces from sunlight or absorbs from milk is inactivated and needs to be converted into calcitriol in the liver and kidneys. If the body has insufficient levels of parathyroid hormones, which aid this process, then supplementation with activated vitamin D may be necessary.

Not only do I have to worry about my calcium level dropping too low, but I've also been warned not to let it get too high. Besides aiding in the conversion of vitamin D, parathyroid hormones help the kidneys keep calcium from filtering out of the blood. With insufficient parathyroid levels, too much calcium flows out of the blood, causing the possibility of kidney stones and hypercalciuria [high levels of calcium in the urine]. No drug exists to prevent this.

Over the next several months, I suffered from paresthesias, a burning sensation that felt like a bug crawling on my lips, a lot of twitching, especially in my legs, and some obscure symptoms such as tremors inside my eyeballs, and seizures in my tongue and nose. Even though I was taking large amounts of calcium and Rocaltrol, I still suffered. I spent a lot of time asking my colleague questions like: what were her symptoms after surgery; how long did it take her body to stabilize; did she still have symptoms while taking medication; how long before she develops symptoms if she forgets to take her medication, etc.

At first I wanted to hear stories about people whose temporary hypocalcemia disappeared, who were able to get off their medication, but as time wore on, I realized I had a permanent problem. I didn't want to hear any more about the "lucky" ones. It wasn't fair.

It took a long time to determine the right dosage. I started off taking calcium carbonate (Tums Ultra), but switched to calcium citrate after discovering that high blood alkaline levels contribute to twitching. Calcium citrate is slightly more expensive, but has been found to be a more absorbable form of calcium. It can be taken with or without food. Although it has been documented that the body can only absorb 500 mg of calcium (Ca) at a time, I don't think a study has been done on people taking Rocaltrol. I take 1,000 mg calcium morning and night, along with Rocaltrol. It's also been documented that calcium levels are negatively affected by foods high in phosphates, something I keep in mind.

My parathyroid problems bothered me for a long time. It was an emotional roller coaster. I couldn't get away from the twitching and it drove me to distraction. At one point, I was thinking about timing the seconds between twitches because I was sure that I had a twitch somewhere in my body every 30 seconds.

4
MEDULLARY THYROID CANCER

As discussed in chapter 1, there is a type of thyroid cancer called medullary cancer, which accounts for less than one out of 10 cases found in the U.S. each year. Roughly one third of patients with medullary thyroid cancer have inherited a defective (mutant) gene which causes this cancer and may be passed on to other family members. The other people with this cancer, develop medullary thyroid cancer without having an inherited gene [mutation].

The thyroid gland contains two major types of thyroid cells. One type, the follicular cell, is the cell that is able to take up iodine and make thyroid hormone; turning into a papillary or follicular thyroid cancer in the event of it transforming into cancer. The other type is the parafollicular cell (also known as the "C cell" and located near the thyroid follicular cells) which makes several other hormones and proteins, including calcitonin. The parafollicular cell can become transformed into a medullary thyroid cancer, sometimes because of an inherited gene mutation (the mutation is called "RET proto-oncogene mutation"). If you or a family member are found to have a medullary thyroid cancer, a blood test is performed to evaluate the genes for this mutation. If this mutation is found, then blood tests of other family members may reveal this mutation in them. In previous years, blood tests for calcitonin were performed; however these tests were not very sensitive, had to be repeated every year, and often missed the opportunity to detect this cancer before it had spread.

Medullary thyroid cancer can often be very slow-growing, but is considered potentially very dangerous because there aren't any effective ways to treat this cancer if it spreads outside of the neck. Sometimes it can be more aggressive and grow more rapidly, spreading to many parts of the body. The "RET proto-oncogene test" has been extremely important in helping with this cancer. If you test positive for this inherited medullary thyroid cancer gene, the recommendation, is to have what's called a "prophylactic thyroidectomy," meaning a preventative removal of the entire thyroid gland. This removes the risk of ever developing medullary thyroid cancer, which can spread and develop into more serious cancer. In some cases, the cancer has already formed before the surgery is done, although the genetic test permits the treatment to begin sooner than would have happened without it. Unlike other cancers studied with genetic tests, medullary thyroid cancer is unique in that if a mutation is found in the RET proto-oncogene, it is essentially a near certainty that this cancer has developed or will develop. For this reason, thyroid cancer specialists recommend this surgery as soon as possible. It is standard practice for children with this gene to have this surgery as soon as they are at least two to five years of age in order to prevent cancers which can begin quite early. In addition to medullary thyroid cancer, some patients with this "RET proto-oncogene mutation" may also inherit a combination of additional problems, the Multiple Endocrine Neoplasia syndromes (see further). These are known as MEN-2A (with overactive parathyroid glands causing elevated calcium levels in the blood and tumors of the adrenal gland causing high levels of adrenaline) or MEN-2B (with the same adrenal tumors and tiny bumps on the tongue and lips).

Signs of Medullary Thyroid Cancer

The signs of medullary thyroid cancer are the same as they are for papillary and follicular, in that a lump may be felt on the thyroid or neck. However, some of medullary thyroid cancer patients will experience diarrhea as a result of the tumor. The diarrhea is actually caused by gastrointestinal secretions and a speeding up of your gastrointestinal nerves and muscles (known as hypermotility). This is thought to occur because the tumor secretes calcitonin, prostaglandins and serotonin. Sudden diarrhea may actually get any primary care doctor thinking "gastrointestinal cancer" rather than thyroid cancer, however. And it could send you off on a wild ride of the wrong tests with gastroenterologists, when what you really need is a thyroid specialist. If you know that you have the gene for inherited medullary thyroid cancer or multiple endocrine neoplasm syndromes (see further), and have not had a prophylactic thyroidectomy, then sudden diarrhea is a sign that you should run—not walk—to a thyroid specialist.

The General Medullary Picture

Medullary thyroid cancer accounts for five to eight percent of all thyroid cancers, and usually starts in the upper center of the thyroid gland. It does not develop in the cells of the thyroid that make thyroid hormone; it develops in the "C cells" (known as as the parafollicular cells), which make the hormone calcitonin, as discussed in the Introduction. Medullary thyroid cancer can grow very slowly, so 10-year survival rates are 90 percent for medullary thyroid cancer confined to the thyroid; however, these cancers can continue to grow and spread over several decades, requiring lifelong screening. The survival rate drops slightly down to 70 percent when it has spread to the lymph nodes in the neck, which tends to happen frequently. If it has spread to other organs, the survival rates plummet to roughly 20 percent and worsen with time. Men over 50 with medullary thyroid cancer tend to have a more aggressive strain of it, which is usually not genetic in origin, and not as good an outcome as women or younger men. Sadly, there are no sensitive methods to scan and detect or treat this type of cancer with radioactive iodine. Instead, recurrence is tracked by measuring levels of calcitonin. Imaging tests are also rarely able to detect the spread of medullary thyroid cancer tumors.

Types of Medullary Thyroid Cancer

Most medullary thyroid cancers develop without having a RET proto-ongogene mutation as their cause and are called "sporadic." Sporadic medullary thyroid cancer is typically diagnosed in women aged 40-60, and less commonly in men. This type of medullary thyroid cancer is usually diagnosed via FNA (see chapter 2) from a lump on the thyroid gland or beyond, similar to the way papillary or follicular cancer is diagnosed.

Inherited medullary thyroid cancer is the least aggressive type of medullary cancer and tends to strike in the 40s and 50s.

Multiple Endocrine Neoplasias (MEN)

Here's where it gets *weird*. Medullary thyroid cancer caused by the mutated RET proto-oncogene, can happen as just medullary thyroid cancer, or can happen in combination with other types of hormonal tumors entirely separate from thyroid cancer. Known as multiple endocrine neoplasia syndromes or "MEN" (pronounced by spelling out "M," "E," "N,"), these are endocrine syndromes that comprise different "packages" of diseases, all occurring at once. Quite the nightmare, actually. So...

Medullary thyroid cancer can occur as part of the package known as "Sipple syndrome" or "MEN-2A." This disease "package" comes equipped with: medullary thyroid cancer; a condition known as pheochromocytoma, where tumors on the adrenal glands cause you to overproduce stress hormones known as epinephrine and norepinephrine, producing a "flight or fight" response and panic attacks (see chapter 8); and hyperparathyroidism (opposite of hypoparathyroidism) in which the parathyroid glands make too much parathyroid hormone, causing increased levels of calcium. The RET proto-oncogene mutation in MEN-2A is a "dominant" inherited trait, meaning that the chance is 50/50 that any child of such a person would also get this mutation and get this package of problems.

The next "package" is called MEN-2B. This comes equipped with: medullary thyroid cancer; pheochromocytoma, and a combination of one or more of mucosal ganglioneuromas (lumpy, bumpy lips and tongue), an unusual body type characterized by long fingers and toes, (which resembles a body type seen with a syndrome known as Marfan's syndrome), and thickened nerves in the cornea of the eyes. Lastly, some inherited medullary thyroid cancers do not have other unusual features of MEN-2A or MEN-2B, although they are caused by similar "RET proto-oncogene" mutations.

Staging and Spreading

As in papillary and follicular thyroid cancer, medullary thyroid cancer can be diagnosed in different stages. Stage I means the tumor is less than one centimeter in size and is confined to the thyroid. Stage II means the tumor is larger than one in size, but is confined to the thyroid. Stage III means the cancer has spread to the lymph nodes in the neck. Stage IV means the cancer has spread to other parts of the body beyond the neck.

Treatment Options

Because medullary thyroid cancer is unable to be easily treated once it is outside of the thyroid's region, a total thyroidectomy and neck dissection is recommended. These procedures are discussed in chapter 3. Radioactive iodine does not tend to have an effect on medullary thyroid cancer and is therefore not part of the treatment scenario. But because medullary thyroid cancer can be followed by detecting calcitonin levels in the blood, this is an excellent method to track recurrence. Levels of a protein known as carcinoembryonic antigen (CEA), also made by the parafollicular cells in the thyroid, can be tracked through a blood test as well, and is used for the same purpose. External beam radiation (discussed in chapter 7) may also be offered for any of the stages, depending upon recurrence, although this is very controversial, while chemotherapy (discussed in the next chapter) is not an option, due to the lack of effective drugs for this type of cancer or stage IV. However, in this case, clinical trials may offer meaningful treatments.

The post-treatment side effects of thyroidectomy, such as hypothyroidism, are discussed in chapter 3. Although you'll be placed on thyroid hormone replacement to compensate for hypothyroidism, there is no need, in this case, to be put on a TSH-suppression dosage of thyroid hormone, since medullary thyroid cancer is *not* affected by thyroid stimulating hormone. Thyroid medication is discussed in chapter 7.

Genetic Screening for Family Members

Not all medullary thyroid cancer is inherited; indeed, most of it occurs sporadically, without any genetic cause. But since three types of medullary thyroid cancer are inherited, it's a good idea to discuss genetic screening with other family members. If multiple endocrine neoplasm syndromes run in your family, you are at risk for medullary thyroid cancer. Similary, if inherited medullary thyroid cancer runs in your family, you are also at risk.

Generally first-degree relatives (e.g., siblings and children) are more at risk for inherited medullary thyroid cancer than more distant relatives (such as aunts and cousins). In chapter 1, there is a discussion about the benefits of genetic testing for this type of cancer. Review that section if you decide you want to be screened for the medullary thyroid cancer gene. Since there is a way to absolutely prevent inherited medullary thyroid cancer (through total thyroidectomy), while the gene causing it almost guarantees the development of this type of cancer, genetic screening in this case has more clear benefits than genetic screening for other types of cancers such as breast or colon, which are triggered by environmental factors.

Prophylactic Thyroidectomy

If you've come from a family where someone has the inherited form of medullary thyroid cancer, or you've tested positive for the gene mutation yourself, you definitely ought to consider what's called a prophylactic total thyroidectomy (meaning you have your thyroid removed before it's clinically necessary) to prevent the development of medullary thyroid cancer in the future. The risks of this are the same as those outlined in chapter 3; in addition, you'll become permanently hypothyroid and will have to be on lifelong medication via thyroid hormone replacement.

Calcitonin Screening for Recurrence

If you've been treated for medullary thyroid cancer with a total thyroidectomy, you won't have many C cells left to secrete calcitonin. Therefore, a blood test that detects calcitonin is a sign that the cancer has recurred. You should be followed up, therefore, with a regular blood test that checks for any detectable levels of calcitonin.

5

ANAPLASTIC THYROID CANCER AND OTHER UNRESPONSIVE AGGRESSIVE TUMORS

Anaplastic thyroid cancer accounts for a paltry 1.6 percent of *all* thyroid cancers, which translates into about 300 cases in the United States per year. However, it is an aggressive, *wildly undifferentiated* cancer that has no real cure. This chapter will give you the true facts about your options for quality of life for the remaining time you have. It's important to plan for the present, because the outcomes are so dismal in this case. Less than one percent of people diagnosed with anaplastic thyroid cancer are even alive beyond two years. Dr. Kenneth Ain, a thyroid cancer specialist on the Medical Advisory Board of the Thyroid Cancer Survivor's Association (Thyca), stated in 2000 that when he sees a patient who has lived one year after being diagnosed with anaplastic thyroid cancer, he believes that patient has been misdiagnosed and, in fact, has a different cancer, such as lymphoma.

Anaplastic thyroid cancer is a mutation of a pre-existing papillary or follicular cancer and does not just sprout by itself, although it can take roughly 20 years to really develop. It's diagnosed, like papillary and follicular, from lumps or usually from a growing mass in the neck region. Physical signs of anaplastic cancer include hoarseness, shortness of breath, and difficulty swallowing—symptoms associated with cancerous growths on the trachea. More than 95 percent of anaplastic thyroid cancers spread distantly, through the bloodstream to sites in the lung, liver, bones, and brain. Fifty percent of all anaplastic thyroid cancer is diagnosed after it's already spread to the lung. Because it takes so long to develop, it is usually seen in people 65 and older, and women are diagnosed with it twice as often as men. About four to 10 percent of anaplastic thyroid cancer is diagnosed in people under 50.

When you're diagnosed with anaplastic thyroid cancer, you're really being diagnosed with a much more known disease in the cancer world: *metastatic disease.* That's what you should be looking up on the Internet as your "keyword." According to the top experts in anaplastic thyroid cancer, the major approach to treatment involves prolonging your life and using various therapies discussed below to allow for a comfortable quality of life for as long as possible. This involves treating the primary tumor (the thyroid gland site) aggressively, with as complete surgical removal as possible, followed by high-dose external beam radiotherapy to the neck. Although everyone will eventually succumb to metastatic disease, without surgery to remove the growing thyroid cancers, strangulation can occur.

Some surgeons perform a tracheostomy, which involves taking out part of the tube through which a person breathes, and replacing it with a plastic one, but anaplastic thyroid cancer experts maintain that there's no evidence that this is useful as a routine procedure for anaplastic thyroid cancer and most patients do better without it.

There's almost no meaningful research or information on anaplastic cancer treatment available online or at medical libraries. You'll read that if it's "diagnosed early" (which almost never occurs), a total thyroidectomy and neck dissection (see chapter 3), followed by external beam radiation therapy (see chapter 6), followed by chemotherapy, is the treatment. But all meaningful treatment protocols are being done through clinical trials that are currently unpublished. It may be useful to visit *www.clinicaltrials.gov* or *http://cancernet.nci.nih.gov/trialsrch.shtml* to ask about clinical trials. But when you're talking about a cancer that makes up only 1.6 percent of all thyroid cancers (which generally occur in only one percent of the entire population anyway), you're not likely to find too many clinical trials going on for anaplastic thyroid cancer. The shortest route is to contact the University of Kentucky Medical Center, which has ongoing clinical trials in anaplastic thyroid cancer through its thyroid nodule and oncology clinic. You might also find meaningful trials to treat metastatic disease. In essence, having anaplastic thyroid cancer means that you have metastatic disease. Instead of thinking about "treatment" you need to focus on "quality of life" options.

What Is Metastatic Disease?

Metastatic disease means the cancer has spread to other organs in the body. And the cancer is now systemic, meaning it is involving several organ systems at once. It's a term used to describe the spread of any advanced cancer. Symptoms of metastatic disease include:

1. Dry, persistent cough. This indicates a problem with the lungs.
2. Difficulty breathing or shortness of breath. Again, this indicates a problem with the lungs.
3. General aches and pains or stiffness. This can indicate that the cancer has spread to the bones.
4. Enlarged lymph nodes—anywhere! Lymph nodes under the arms, neck, collar bone area and groin area should be checked regularly. Immediately report any enlargement to your doctor.
5. General fatigue. This is a sign that you're fighting off something. It could be the flu; it could be cancer. Report this to your doctor.
6. Sores that don't heal or rashes—especially in the upper body region.
7. Changes in weight or appetite and/or fevers. This is a sign of a possible problem with the liver.
8. Headaches and/or vision problems that get progressively worse with time. These are signs of cancer in the brain or eye region. However, having a headache can just mean you have a headache!
9. Muscle weakness or paralysis. This can be a sign of brain or spinal cord metastasis.
10. Extreme, localized pain along your spinal column. This is a sign of metastasis to the spinal cord—not a common site, however.

To Treat or Not to Treat?

As discussed earlier, many of you may want to consider entering experimental clinical trials (known as Phase I trials), which offer the chance of benefiting from a new and untested treatment, as well as better care and attention. At the same time, it may also be worth considering whether entering the trial has other risks attached. In other words, is being treated worth it? Here are some key questions that can determine whether it's worth it:

1. How many places has the cancer spread? Obviously, the less, the better. If it's throughout your body, you're probably better off looking at palliative care and pain management.

2. Which sites have cancer? Cancers tend to multiply faster in the liver, but slower in bone.

3. How severe are your symptoms? If you can barely breathe, something like radiation therapy may be used to shrink the size of tumors for optimal comfort, while no symptoms may warrant a different approach.

4. What is your overall health? Chemotherapy may be too harsh if you're elderly and too frail for the side effects.

5. How will treatment affect your day-to-day life? Questions revolving around fatigue and traveling to the treatment's location, etc. are all valid. Find out!

6. Will this treatment prolong your life (if so, by how much)? In the final analysis, are you gaining anything or just losing valuable time?

7. What are the short-term side effects of this treatment? Nausea, vomiting and hair loss are an example of "short-term" side effects.

8. Is this treatment covered by my insurer? If you lose your insurance coverage over not-very-tangible benefits, you may want to reconsider. (Not a concern for Canadians.)

9. How will this treatment affect my immune system? This is a crucial question. Chemotherapy, in particular, will suppress your immune system, leaving you vulnerable to infections and viruses you may never have had before.

Other factors to consider are the goals of the treatment, and the extent to which you want treatment. Many people with metastatic disease choose alternative therapies (see chapter 9) over more aggressive Western therapies. Many people opt for palliative care in conjunction with alternative healing. (Palliative care is discussed in the next section.) So treatment will vary depending on the desired outcome: cure or prolonged survival (if a cure isn't possible); relief of symptoms or maintaining quality of life for as long as possible.

If you have no symptoms, you may decide to carry on with life as before and live it to the fullest. After all, having cancer doesn't mean you're *suddenly* mortal; it simply means you're facing mortality sooner than the person who gets killed suddenly in a car accident. No treatment is certainly a worthwhile consideration when you consider the side effects of treatment are sometimes worse than the disease itself.

Attitude is everything in this case. No matter which cancer expert or survivor you speak to, the overwhelming majority reports that attitude counts. This is one reason why so many Western practitioners are welcoming the addition of complementary therapies (see chapter 9). These span from dietary adjustments, herbal and vitamin supplements to therapeutic massage, breathing, and meditating. Thyroid cancer specialists maintain that taking a leap of faith from your own traditions and cultures into belief systems that are foreign to you is not necessary in terms of fostering a "good attitude." Turning to your own belief systems and support networks instead of trying to "learn a new religion" in order to prolong your life is what being positive means. It's also important to note that many people waste good quality time with family and friends by "rainbow chasing" wild and untested alternative cancer therapies, which for the most part are never designed as curative, but rather complementary to overall health and well-being. Yoga, for example, will not cure your cancer; however, it can help you find peace and tranquility.

Cancer survivors also report that the actual day-to-day confrontation with one's mortality is strangely healing. Many report living with a heightened awareness as well as with less stress because they are living the essential life, rather than a life burdened with trivial worries.

Treating Metastatic Disease with Chemotherapy

Chemotherapy was an accidental discovery that grew out of troops' exposure to mustard gas during both world wars. Although mustard gas wasn't officially used in World War II, it was during *this* war that the medicinal benefits of mustard gas became obvious. After a ship carrying the gas was bombed in an Italian harbor, survivors of the blast showed a dramatic drop in white blood cells—something that's bad news for healthy people, but good news for people with leukemia. The rest is history. Chemotherapy soon became standard treatment for leukemia, presenting the first possibilities for a cure. Within a couple of decades leukemia treatment formed the basis for many cancer treatments: using poisonous agents to kill cancer cells.

Chemotherapy is a pretty universal experience for all cancer patients, possibly with the exception of other thyroid cancer patients you may meet! In other words, whether you're having chemo for anaplastic thyroid cancer, ovarian cancer, leukemia or breast cancer, the experience is the same.

Chemotherapy simply means treating some kind of medical condition with drugs. So technically, taking Aspirin or antibiotics are both forms of chemotherapy. When it comes to cancer, you're taking *anti-cancer drugs*. These drugs are designed to kill cancer cells. They interfere with the process of cell division or reproduction so that the cells can't divide and, therefore, will die. But the drugs are not very selective and kill *healthy* cells that are also dividing, including hair cells and bone marrow cells.

Basically the line between a therapeutic dosage and a toxic dosage is quite fine, and for this reason, only a highly experienced medical oncologist is qualified to manage your chemotherapy. Chemotherapy drugs can be administered orally or intravenously. You might be given just one kind of drug, or a combination of drugs. Combination drug therapy is often done because most chemotherapy drugs are not always effective when used individually, so multiple drugs are used to overcome drug resistance. Each drug comes with its own list of potential side effects. Drugs that were once commonly used to treat anaplastic thyroid cancer include doxirubicin, 5-fluorouracil (called 5-FU), vincristine sulfate, cisplatin, and bleomycin. But more recent studies show that paclitaxel (Taxol) is the most effective chemotherapy drug for anaplastic thyroid cancer, as well as the best tolerated.

Pharmacists recommend getting information from the United States Pharmacopeia Drug Information (USP DI) or the American Society of Hospital Pharmacists book of drug information for consumers. In Canada, the *Compendium of Pharmaceuticals and Specialties* (CPS) would have this information. Many pharmacies now offer extensive drug information for patients as an added value service. Another option is to look up your drug in a *pharmaceutical compendium*, such as the *Physician's Desk Reference* (in libraries) for the complete story, however this information is very technical and may not be suitable for the lay public. I recommend getting this information prior to starting your drug therapy so you can review it with your doctor and be fully prepared.

There are general side effects common to all of the anti-cancer drugs, however. That's because no matter how balanced your chemotherapy dosage is, your healthy cells will be affected. Reactions *do* vary from person to person, and there are certain medications, such as anti-nausea drugs, for example, that are often added to your therapy to reduce the infamous vomiting and nausea.

Some of the more common reactions to chemo include: tiredness, weakness, body aches, bloating and weight gain, night sweats, nausea, loss of appetite and changes in your sense of taste and smell (you may notice a chemical odor all the time, for instance). It's not uncommon to have mouth sores, dry mouth, pink eye (conjunctivitis), "allergy symptoms" (watery eyes and runny nose), bleeding gums and headaches, as well as diarrhea and constipation. Less common are tingling fingers and toes, and a loss of muscle strength. Some or all of the above may be mild, moderate or severe, and you can be given medications to relieve many of these symptoms.

Chemo can also cause a chemically induced depression (charmingly known as "chemo brain"), and can cause dramatic mood swings. Hair loss (clinically known as alopecia) is the classic side effect, but the most serious one is immune suppression, which can leave you vulnerable to a host of viruses. Other side effects include a decrease in your blood *platelets*, which are responsible for blood clotting. You might find that you're bruising easily, bleed more when you're cut, or bleed suddenly out of your nose or even rectum. This will improve after your treatment, but please report your bleeding episodes to your doctor so your dosage can be adjusted if necessary.

If you experience any of the following symptoms, notify your doctor immediately. This is a sign that you may need to stop the chemotherapy NOW!

- Severe diarrhea.
- Severe stomach pains (a sign of gastritis—inflammation of your stomach lining).
- Dry cough (without sputum or mucus)—a sign of a possible lung infection.
- An active infection or virus (flu-like symptoms and fever should be reported).
- Fever (especially if accompanied by a dry cough).
- Shortness of breath.

Treating Metastatic Disease with Radiation

In metastatic disease, radiation therapy is often used as a symptom reliever. Because it can shrink tumors, this can relieve the pressure from a number of areas, which is often the reason why you're experiencing pain. If your cancer has spread to the bone, radiation is particularly helpful because it can shrink the tumor and relieve the pressure in the bone, preventing further bone damage.

Radiation is also more effective for bone pain because the bone can tolerate far higher doses of radiation than other parts of the body and because pain is often effectively relieved by radiation. Bones, unlike many parts of the body, can be treated with radiation more than once.

Treating fluid accumulation

This is a condition that often occurs when cancer spreads to the lungs and blocks the lymph nodes that drain the area. Fluid begins to accumulate, causing shortness of breath and sharp chest pain—especially when breathing deeply.

If you have these symptoms, a physical exam and chest x-ray will confirm the diagnosis. The treatment is to drain the fluid by inserting a tube into the chest. Antibiotics are also used to help fight off infection in the area.

Sometimes fluid can accumulate in the abdomen, which causes swelling and bloat. Ultrasound and a physical exam will confirm the problem, and a catheter is inserted into the abdomen to drain the fluid.

Palliative Care

Palliative care refers to symptom relief, and is a component of all medical care, whether the intent is to cure a disease or to eliminate its symptoms. People at all stages of an illness will want to be free of spiritual, psychological and physical symptoms from the earliest stage of diagnosis until they are cured, or die. But what does it mean to treat the *symptoms* of a disease, rather than the disease itself? What it sometimes boils down to is different goals.

Whenever anyone needs medicine or therapies to relieve the pain or symptoms of any given illness, it's known as "palliative care." Palliative care generally enters into the cancer picture in a situation where metastatic disease has developed and there are no therapies available that can cure the disease. In this case, the goals of therapy change from what doctors call a curative approach, meaning that therapies and medications are designed to cure the cancer, to a palliative approach, where medications and therapies are designed not to cure, but to make you comfortable and alert so you can carry on as normally as possible.

Your thyroid specialist can refer you to a palliative care team at your medical center, which may consist of several consulting doctors, nurses, physiotherapist, pharmacist, psychologist, social worker, clergy, dietitian, and volunteers. Palliative care can also be "portable." Although you may be hospitalized, depending on your health you may also be able to receive treatment as an outpatient through regular visits to the hospital or your palliative care specialist.

You have the right to expect the following from your palliative care team:

1. An open-ended approach to therapy. In other words, your care should be flexible to meet your changing needs rather than rigid and finite.

2. No blanket reassurances that everything will be fine. Your team should be frank about your prognosis but sensitive to your feelings.

3. As much information as you want, whenever you want it.

4. Jargon-free explanations. This means non-technical descriptions of what's happening in your body, and non-technical descriptions of the therapy recommended to relieve symptoms.

5. Ongoing assessment. You should be regularly assessed by your doctor and informed about your illness' progression and symptoms to expect. In this case, your health may be changing daily.

6. Participation in your treatment.

7. The goals of your treatment defined in black and white. For example, if you're having radiation therapy to your chest area to shrink a tumor, the goal is "to shrink the tumor so you can breathe more easily"—not to cure the cancer.

8. Techniques for coping with family and friends. You should be able to count on your team for supportive advice in dealing with family or friends who are in conflict or denial about your situation.

The Symptoms You're Palliating

One of the most common symptoms of metastatic disease is shortness of breath. This has a number of causes ranging from fluid accumulation, which can be removed; pneumonia, which can be treated with antibiotics; hyperventilation due to anxiety, relieved through breathing techniques or anti-anxiety medications; or a tumor pressing down on the lungs, which may require you to be on oxygen at home or in the hospital. As a final step, if there's no way to remove the cause of shortness of breath, narcotics such as morphine or hydromorphine will decrease the *sensation* of breathlessness.

Loss of appetite (called "anorexia") is another common symptom associated with advanced cancer. Sometimes this has to do with where your cancer is located; other times it's a response to pain medication. The most upsetting aspect of appetite loss is what it does it to the people around you. So the first rule is to have your palliative team reassure your family and friends that food is not a guarantee of a longer life span. Generally, dietitians recommend that you have people prepare foods in very small portions—"single-wrapped" or "finger food" formats. You'll find food much more appetizing this way. Meal replacement drinks can also solve some problems. You can sip on a can or two throughout the day, which will still be packed with a fair bit of calories and vitamins.

Mild to severe nausea is also a symptom in advanced cancer, which is either a result of your cancer or a response to various medications. The solutions here vary from anti-nausea medications to adjusting diet or medications accordingly.

On the flip side, you may also be constipated, a classic symptom of narcotic pain relief, which can be alleviated with laxatives and stool softeners. Bladder incontinence can be another symptom, which can be alleviated with either a catheter or bladder control undergarments.

Fatigue strikes again with advanced cancer. Fatigue in this case is often a sign that you're not sleeping well at night because your pain is waking you up. This means that you need a stronger pain control medication, discussed further on. Fatigue can, of course, be a side effect of treatments such as radiation and narcotic medications like codeine or morphine.

Pain Management

You can be seriously ill without severe physical pain and require nothing more than some over-the-counter drugs. However, when advanced cancer causes severe pain, you're going to need some strong stuff to control it. Your doctor will usually start with a non-narcotic and work his/her way up to a narcotic painkiller, known as an "opioid" (the root word comes from opium—one of the oldest narcotics). Narcotic medication for severe pain control is generally not addictive in the sense that you don't wait for your next "fix" so you can become "strung out" on drugs. There are also many narcotics that now come in pain patches (worn on the skin like nicotine patches), which eliminate much of the dosage administering of days gone by.

What happens, though, is that when the drug wears off, you'll feel the pain again, so you'll want another dose just to feel *normal*. And that's fine. That's what a narcotic is designed to do.

So while narcotics may be a godsend, they're still, of course, power-ful drugs that you can't just take by yourself when you feel like it. You're going to need someone who is an expert at administering the lowest pos-sible dose of a narcotic, based on a number of factors: where your pain is located; the cause of your pain; how much pain you have; and your over-all health. But patients and their families are being encouraged by spe-cialists to become their own gauge in managing and administering their narcotic dosages.

Pain is a sign that something's wrong. You already know that now, but your body doesn't *know* you do. In the same way that your smoke detec-tor will continue to ring until the smoke clears, your body will continue to send pain signals until you remove the cause of the pain. Until that day comes (which is probably unlikely in advanced cancer), you have to *deaden* the pain. Your nerve endings act as the "smoke detectors" in your body. Every part of your body has free nerve endings, while the spinal cord has pain receptors, which tell your brain to tell those nerve endings to send the pain.

Sometimes it's the nerves themselves that are damaged, due to nerve compression or compression of the spinal cord. This will cause that inter-mittent, stabbing pain, often accompanied by a burning or numbness. Other times pain is caused by tumors that infiltrate bone or press down on other organs. This will lead to more continuous, aching pain.

Pain has many shapes and forms, which will help tell your pallia-tive care team what's going on. For example, you can have acute pain, which means that the pain has a clear beginning, middle, and end. Acute pain also has physical signs, such as a sweating, pupil dilation, and a pounding heart.

Chronic pain is harder to describe because it goes on and on in a con-tinuous aching. It's difficult for your doctors to tell sometimes when you have chronic pain because people may describe it as "discomfort" or "unwellness." In others, chronic pain triggers depression, irritability or sleeplessness. Or, as your illness advances and you become more debili-tated, depressed or anxious about your circumstance, your awareness of pain increases, which will make the pain feel worse (even though it may actually be the same pain you've been dealing with for a while).

There's another condition known as "total pain." This is when you're just "maxxed out" from a variety of pains related to your illness: pain from the disease itself; side effects of your treatment or medications; emo-tional pain, and so on. It's the equivalent of pain "burnout."

The number one goal of pain management in cancer is to either prevent or completely control pain. Period. No exceptions. So the first thing your doctor will do is try to figure out what's causing your pain. For example, if a tumor is pressing down on an organ, it can often be shrunk with radiation, or surgically removed, which will then eliminate the pain without resorting to narcotic drugs.

Your doctor will also try get you to assess your pain on a number system from zero to five. Zero = no pain; one = mild; two = discomforting; three = distressing; four = horrible; and five = excruciating. This will tell your doctor what type of medications you need for pain control. Obviously a five will require the "hard stuff" while a two or three may be able to be managed with a non-narcotic medication.

Drugs That Control Pain

There are classes of drugs used to control pain, which doctors prescribe in a "stepped care" approach. That means they start with the least powerful drug and work their way up as the pain increases.

On the bottom step is a class of drugs known as non-opioids (a.k.a. non-narcotics). These are basic pain killers (analgesics) such as acetylsalicylic acid or A.S.A.(Aspirin), acetaminophen (Tylenol) and non-steroidal anti-inflammatory drugs (NSAIDs), such as ibuprofen or naproxen (Naprosyn). These drugs work by interfering with body chemicals called *prostaglandins*, which normally cause inflammation and increase your body's pain receptor "firing." Non-narcotics are used not just for mild pain, but also for bone pain and other forms of severe pain.

The second step up the pain ladder is what's called a weak opioid, which is often mixed with a non-opioid. A weak opioid is codeine, and it's often mixed with acetaminophen in a drug such as Tylenol #3. The third and final step up is a strong opioid. This is when morphine or hydromorphone is used. Both weak and strong opioids are known as narcotics. These work in the central nervous system (the brain and spinal cord), and inhibit the transmission of pain. Most narcotics used in advanced cancer treatment are morphine preparations and hydromorphine (Dilaudid). Less common are propoxyphene (Darvon), oxycodone (Percodan), and oxymorphone (Numorphan).

Co-analgesics

On every step in the pain management ladder, your doctor may decide to combine your analgesic with a drug that will relieve other symptoms of your illness, or prevent the side effects of your painkiller. For example, anticonvulsants, antidepressants, steroids, membrane stabilizing drugs or anti-anxiety drugs may all be added to non-opioids, weak or strong opioids.

Taking drugs "as needed" vs. round-the-clock

As discussed, depending on the kind of pain you have, your doctor will want to prevent it or control it. To prevent pain, you'll be on what's called a "regular" dosing schedule whether you have pain or not. This is better than waiting for the pain to build up and much less stressful for you. In this case, however, you must take the dose as prescribed; no more drug, no less drug, taken no more or less frequently than prescribed. Otherwise, either the pain will not be managed properly or else too much of the drug will build up in your system so that it becomes toxic to your general health.

Taking medications "as needed," (known as p.r.n. in PharmacySpeak) is a little trickier. You must take the drug as soon as you start to feel the least bit uncomfortable. If you wait until the pain increases (in an effort to "tough it out" until it gets really bad), the drug just won't work as well, and you'll have to take higher doses. Of course, it may well be that you don't need to be on as high a dose of the drug as you are, or that another drug may work better. So be on the lookout for "post-dose" symptoms such as agitation or extreme drowsiness. This may mean that your doctor needs to adjust the dosage or switch the drug.

So long as your doctor knows what's causing your pain, you should be able to have as much analgesia as you need to control the pain. In fact, nurses on palliative care wards in hospitals should have standing orders to increase your pain medication if it's not strong enough.

Dosing is another issue around narcotics. There is no standard or *maximum* dose for these medications. Dosing varies on the individual situation—and the individual. So it's important for you or your family (if you're not able) to keep a diary of when you're experiencing pain so you and your doctor can develop a regular dosing schedule that prevents what's called "breakthrough pain."

Balancing your medications is another issue, particularly when co-analgesics (see above) are added to your pain medications. Ask your doctor or pharmacist to draw up a chart that you can follow listing all the medications you need to take and when you need to take them. It's usually fine to take all your various medications as a "group" (i.e., analgesic, antidepressant and narcotic) in the morning, for example, and then at other times in the day as prescribed. This is easier than taking, say, your analgesic at 8:00 am, your antidepressant at 10:00 am and your narcotic at noon, repeating this a second or third time. That's enough to confuse anybody!

Constipation, discussed briefly above, is a major side effect with narcotics, aggravated by less fluid and food intake and less mobility. Again, laxatives and stool softeners should be combined with any narcotic medication you're on.

If You're Not Finding Relief

Most people do best with a combination of prescription and over-the-counter painkillers. Specialists usually encourage their patients to manage painkillers on their own as much as possible. Since you are, after all, the one experiencing your pain, it's presumed that you should be more expert on your pain than anyone else. If you're not finding relief, however, it may be a case of inappropriate administration, rather than an ineffective narcotic. Is the doctor prescribing the drug regularly, around-the-clock? Is the drug's duration of action matched to its dosing schedule? In other words, if the drug lasts for two hours, but is only being prescribed every four, you'll be in pain for two hours in between! That's *not* a proper way for a painkiller to be administered. In addition, you may simply need a stronger dose of a drug, which is why it's not effective.

Ironically, the longer you're made to wait for another dosage of the drug, the more pain you'll feel out of anticipation and stress. Worse, you're more likely to feel dependent on it and "clock watch" when you're forced to wait for relief.

What You Shouldn't Worry about

A common concern is for palliative care patients to think that large doses of narcotics will mean even larger doses in the future. This isn't true. Once your doctor finds the right dose of narcotic to successfully manage your pain (which can take a few tries), you shouldn't need a dosage increase unless your pain increases—not because you've gotten too used to the narcotic, but because your disease is progressing. But this doesn't mean that you'll ever find your pain is *not* controllable—a very common fear.

Dependence or addiction is another fear that really shouldn't concern you if the drug is being administered appropriately.

Issues Surrounding End of Life

If you're in poor health, at some point you'll need to decide whether you want to be treated at home or in a hospital, or somewhere in between—such as a hospice. What factors into this decision is the availability of homecare or a caregiver, equipment such as an adjustable bed, bedside pans, IV lines, comfort devices such as special mattresses, hand rails, mechanical aids for bath/shower, oxygen and suction equipment, walkers, chairs, wheelchairs, and so on. If you're currently hospitalized, you can request an overnight pass and try going home for a night to see whether your family is able to give you the kind of care you require. This is one way to experiment with different arrangements.

Sometimes the solution is to go for *respite care*, meaning temporary hospital stays to give your family some time off from ongoing caregiving, or to give a paid caregiver time off. Temporary hospital stays can last from one to two weeks.

When it comes to palliative care, more and more hospitals are encouraging patients to receive their care at home. In some cases this is a response to escalating costs; in other cases it's a response to a decrease in the number of beds available. At any rate, it's important to make sure that you're in an environment with:

- Proper equipment and resources.
- Access to ongoing assessment.
- Access to proper symptom and pain control.
- Access to caregiver "substitutes" to relieve caregiver exhaustion.
- Access to emergency care in the case of a problem.

6

RADIOACTIVE WHAT?

As discussed throughout this book, radioactive iodine (RAI) can be selectively taken up, or absorbed by thyroid cancer cells, and is able to be used as a "tracer," lighting up areas of the body with thyroid cancer when viewed on a nuclear medicine scanning camera. It's used to evaluate both thyroid cancer as well as other thyroid problems. Preparing for follow-up scans involves going on a low iodine diet (LID), and either going off thyroid hormone replacement to increase the body's own natural thyroid stimulating hormone (TSH), called a "withdrawal scan", or taking artificially-produced human TSH (Thyrogen®) to stimulate RAI uptake in thyroid cancer cells without the necessity of becoming hypothyroid.

It also involves some degree of isolation of yourself from others until the radioactivity clears from your body. Many of you will also take RAI as a follow-up treatment for thyroid cancer *after* surgery, which also involves being isolated because of the radioactivity. I'll explain all of this in chapter 7. *This* chapter focuses on giving you a thorough explanation of what RAI is, and dispels some myths associated with its use. Obviously, the mere thought of putting RAI into your body is disturbing. Because newly diagnosed thyroid cancer patients are often so "freaked out" over RAI, I felt it necessary to have a "calm down—here's what this stuff is" chapter before launching into the complicated regimens associated with RAI scanning and therapy. The other reason thyroid cancer patients "freak out" over RAI is because of the ridiculous things they hear from ignorant family doctors or other specialists about RAI. I have had thyroid cancer patients call me from all over North America, convinced that they're going to die from leukemia if they take RAI just as a tracer. (That's the most common myth.) If you have medullary thyroid cancer or anaplastic thyroid cancer you won't be offered RAI for follow-up scans or treatment. If you have Hurthle cell thyroid tumors, RAI should be offered because there are no known reasonable alternative treatments for this cancer, although it might not work since some Hurthle cell tumors don't pick up much RAI.

What Is It?

The most frightening aspect of radioactive iodine (RAI) is that it's a very complicated substance to both explain and understand. One must be acquainted with atomic physics and biology to fully comprehend its positive medicinal use on the one hand, and the theoretical risks on the other. You don't have to be a nuclear physicist to understand radioactive iodine, but it helps. When writing the first edition of *The Thyroid Sourcebook* in 1992, I actually did a field interview with a physicist just to understand this stuff, particularly ironic for someone who got a "D" in high school physics! I also had to review the history of the atomic bomb and became quite well versed in the Manhattan Project (rent *Fat Man and Little Boy* and you'll actually understand RAI a little better)!

So let's get started. Charmingly known as the "atomic cocktail," radioactive iodine was discovered accidentally in the 1940s as a by-product of research carried out at the atomic laboratory in Oak Ridge, Tennessee. Although it sounds pretty scary, it's simply an unstable form of iodine. The development of nuclear medicine, used to diagnose and treat certain thyroid disorders, is based on the use of radioactive elements and particles for both testing and treatment. "Radioactive" is the adjective used to describe elements containing *unstable* atoms—or atoms that are emitting energy and hence releasing radiation. A radioactive form of any element is called a radioactive isotope, meaning "unstable variety of this element."

Imagine, for example, that you're trying to carry 300 loose ping-pong balls in your arms from one end of a room to the other without dropping any. It's impossible. Inevitably, as you try to balance and juggle the balls, some *will* drop and fall from your grip. Essentially, this is what happens when an element like iodine is radioactive. The iodine atoms can't securely grip the particles in their center. As a result, some of these sub-atomic particles are "released." The element is therefore *unstable*. But unlike the ping-pong balls, when these particles ("energy") hit the "ground" (in this case, living tissue cells), they can damage and kill the cells.

This is why exposure to too many radioactive particles can cause violent sickness and cancer. However, if you're being treated for cancer, radiation and radioactive particles can be used in a positive way. In this case, the goal of the treatment is to deliberately damage your cancer cells and prevent them from reproducing and spreading throughout your body. To treat thyroid cancer, radioactive *iodine* is used because it is the thyroid's nature to actively take up this particular element, as explained in this book's Introduction.

The "Hot" Topic

The burning question most of you have is "how hot can it get?" RAI is measured in curies or Becquerals (an international unit). A "curie" is the unit of measurement used for radioactive energy, named after the famous scientist, Marie Curie. Doses of RAI are given in either millicuries (one thousandth of a curie) or microcuries (one millionth of a curie). A typical tracer dose of RAI is about two to five millicuries. A typical treatment dose of RAI for thyroid cancer ranges from 100 to 200 millicuries. The amount given depends on the aggressiveness of the thyroid cancer, its ability to take up iodine, and how much cancer was removed during surgery. It's important to note that not all thyroid experts agree about how much radioactive iodine is needed to destroy "leftover" thyroid tissue, or remnant tissue. Some people may receive a dose as low as 29 millicuries, which in the past was the maximum outpatient dose one could receive without requiring to stay in isolation in the hospital. Thyroid cancer experts now consider this too small a therapeutic dose. Rather than prescribe RAI doses to save hospitals the expense of isolation, the trend is to provide the most effective treatment, which means that most people ought to expect an RAI treatment dose exceeding 100 millicuries.

After you receive a treatment dose of radioactive iodine, there's enough radioactivity coming off of your body, in the form of radioactive iodine in your sweat and saliva and x-ray energy, to be a potential source of exposure to others. Depending upon the local regulations of your hospital, dosages ranging from 30 to 150 millicuries may require you to be kept in an isolation room at your hospital. The main reason you're isolated is to comply with public policy regulations and reduce exposure of other people to unnecessary radiation, rather than prevent danger to your dog, cat, or husband. Most nuclear medicine specialists find the isolation rules, which you'll read further on, a bit overly restrictive because the actual risks are quite theoretical and unlikely to ever cause harm to others. Radioactive iodine doesn't hang around too long in your body because most of it gets excreted through urine. It doesn't really "stick" to any part of the body aside from the thyroid cancer cells. The effective "half-life" is the time that it takes for one half of the radioactivity to go away. It's a combination of the "physical" half-life (eight days for iodine-131) and the "biological" half-life (under two days for a person after a thyroidectomy). The effective half-life is usually two to three days, and sufficient radiation leaves your body to allow you to go home in one to three days depending on the hospital's policies and the dosage given.

But the myths surrounding RAI have a longer "half-life" than the isotope itself. Here are most of them:

Myth 1: Radioactive iodine causes leukemia

Fact: Even with a single dosage higher than 800 millicuries of radioactive iodine, fewer than one out of 200 people on that extraordinarily high dosage would go on to develop leukemia, which could not be absolutely linked to RAI and might be expected as a risk of this disease in anyone, unrelated to RAI.

Myth 2: Radioactive iodine causes breast cancer

Fact: A study surfaced in 2000, finding an association between women under 40 who had RAI treatment for thyroid cancer and an increased incidence of breast cancer. The study, conducted by Amy Chen, M.D., M.P.H., of the University of Texas M.D. Anderson Cancer Center in Houston, found that women under 40 who had thyroid cancer are more likely to develop breast cancer later in life, compared to women who have not had thyroid cancer. A theory is that breast tissue, like thyroid tissue, traps iodine, and thus radioactive iodine can predispose both normal thyroid and normal breast tissue to cancer. But every day, studies are finding all kinds of things cause breast cancer, ranging from bras to soy sauce! I was concerned about this, too. As a thyroid cancer survivor as well as the author of *The Breast Sourcebook*, now in its second edition, I wrote a long article exploring this topic for *Thyroid USA*, the newsletter put out by the American Foundation for Thyroid Patients. I concluded that there are so many factors that can cause breast cancer, RAI couldn't be established as an absolute link by itself; indeed, 70 percent of all breast cancers are caused by unknown factors. And the majority of breast cancers, thanks to early screening, are usually caught in early, treatable stages. I encourage you to read this article if you're concerned. The article is called "Breast Cancer Fears: A Closer Look at the Thyroid Cancer-Breast Cancer Link."

Thyroid USA (Volume 9, Issue 2, April, 2002). Here's the link: *http://www.thyroidfoundation.org/breastcancerfears.htm*. A lot of women who've read that article have written to me. They ask: What would I do today if I were diagnosed with thyroid cancer? I would make the same choice regarding RAI—I'd save my life today and have RAI. Then I'd be vigilant about doing Breast Self Exam (BSE), just as I am now. For more on breast cancer, consult my book *The Breast Sourcebook*.

Myth 3: Radioactive iodine causes birth defects

Fact: This has been thoroughly studied over the more than half century that RAI has been used and, to date, there's no evidence that RAI treatments cause any birth defects in babies of women who've completed RAI therapy before their pregnancy. On the other hand, you must be absolutely certain that you're *not* pregnant before you're given any dose of RAI, which would go directly to the fetal thyroid gland and cause severe damage to the fetus. This is why all women in childbearing years have pregnancy tests prior to treatment just to make sure. In other words, you'll need to have a pregnancy test even if you're using birth control; even if you've had a tubal ligation and even if you haven't had sex in months. Even nuns have to have pregnancy tests! You can do this yourself; just get a home pregnancy test kit prior to your RAI scan or treatment and be sure. The test checks for the same thing a lab test does; it detects the hormone, hCG, or human chorionic gonadotropin, the hormone the developing embryo secretes. As long as you wait six months after this treatment before trying to conceive, you'll be just fine. (Of course, pregnancy carries other risks that have nothing to do with radioactive iodine.) For more information on pregnancy and thyroid disease, consult *The Thyroid Sourcebook for Women* or *The Pregnancy Sourcebook*, 3rd edition.

Myth 4: Radioactive iodine causes your hair to fall out

Fact: Oh, it does *not*! People say this because they're confusing this treatment with external radiation therapy, which also doesn't cause hair loss unless the scalp is radiated. People may also be confusing this treatment with chemotherapy, which often causes hair loss, and is discussed in chapter 5.

Myth 5: People with seafood allergies cannot have radioactive iodine therapy

Fact: While seafood contains iodine, the allergy to seafood is rarely a reaction to iodine. So people with this allergy usually do fine. The amount of iodine in an average RAI dose for thyroid cancer amounts to less than three micrograms anyway, a fraction of the iodine in a glass of milk. But if you're concerned, see an allergist beforehand.

What Are the Side Effects?

The word "radioactive" makes people think "radiation sickness" when they think about RAI. In fact, there are very few side effects to RAI for most people. I had none, and had it in liquid form; it tasted like water, and I wondered if they really gave me the "hot stuff" since it didn't feel like anything other than water inside me. That said, the following side effects are reported:

- Sore Throat/Hoarseness. (Or swelling under the ears and jaw, which resembles the "mumps.") This is usually due to swollen salivary glands as a result of the radiation. Sucking on sour candy might help prevent this from occurring although this has never been directly tested or studied. The area around the remaining thyroid tissue can also become tender because of dying thyroid cells.
- Nausea/Vomiting. This is usually caused by your own anxiety and stress over the RAI, which can even induce a panic attack. You can take medication to help with this, and see chapter 8 for more information on dealing with anxiety and panic. If you vomit after having RAI, it will have to be cleaned up for you by a special radiation safety team (see further).
- Headache. Could be caused by stress; probably not by RAI. Plain Tylenol without codeine is best.
- Diarrhea. Diarrhea can be caused by nerves and stress. The more frequently you move your bowels, and the looser they are, the more RAI will clear your system. Keep drinking to avoid dehydration and don't attempt to treat your diarrhea until the RAI is cleared from your system (takes about 48 hours—see further). Also try the BRAT diet: bananas, rice, apple sauce and tea.
- Constipation. Constipation is *not* a good thing after RAI. And it may be the state of affairs if you're hypothyroid. If you haven't had a bowel movement after 12 hours, take a laxative (thyroid cancer experts recommend Milk of Magnesia during RAI treatment). An herbal laxative with cascara segrada is highly effective, and although it's a stimulant laxative, it's not as habit forming as others. Taking fiber is not advised.

- Fatigue. Fatigue is a common sign of hypothyroidism, so it may be caused by that rather than the RAI treatment itself. But then, of course, who wouldn't be tired after all this? Isolation is great for resting. If you're fatigued yet can't sleep, try a little lavender oil on your pillow. Herbal supplements such as valerian root or kava root can help with sleep. Or you can take a sleep aid.

Getting Clearance

Large doses, as mentioned above, require you to be isolated in a private hospital room. No visitors should come without a really good reason; in that case, your hospital will have its own specific rules.

All meals, bedding, and towels will be provided; you may be asked to make your own bed to avoid exposing hospital staff. Some people find this time relaxing—especially if life is hectic. It's forced R & R. You should be advised to change into your hospital gear before the RAI is administered; that way you don't have to worry about your clothing being "hot." Have someone bring you to the hospital, change in the room and either hand your clothes to your support person or keep them in a closet in the room. When you're picked up, you can just remove the hospital gown, shower, and change into fresh clothes. The amount of time you spend in the hospital is based on the amount of RAI you were given.

While in the hospital, you may be required to urinate into a special container that fits like a "pottie" over the toilet bowl; alternatively, you may simply be required to use the bathroom in the room and flush twice. Men will be asked to sit down when they urinate to avoid splashes. In other hospitals, staff may check you with a hand-held "dose-meter" or enter your room and check your urine with a Geiger counter to determine the amount of radioactivity released (based on how much RAI you were given). Once your levels of radiation are "safe" enough for others to be exposed to you, you're allowed to go home, so long as you practice your post-treatment precautions for the next 10 days. The reason for these precautions is to prevent the exposure of others through your saliva, sweat, mucus, urine, feces or other bodily secretions, as well as x-rays coming from the RAI still in your body. You should minimize contact with pregnant women or small children because children, infants and fetuses are more sensitive to radiation exposure. You should use non-porous dishes and cutlery, and wash them before others handle them. You should abstain from all sexual activity (including kissing), sleep alone, and wash your linens and clothing separately after use. After a typical laundry cycle, both the clothing and the washing machine are free of radioactivity. You should use a separate hairbrush, comb, towel, and facecloth, as well as a separate toilet paper roll. Using a damp paper tissue, wipe the toilet seat and sink bowl after each use, flushing the tissue down the toilet. After you use the toilet, you should wash your hands carefully and flush two to three times.

If you use the telephone, you must wipe the mouthpiece with a damp tissue after use. Showering two or three times a day as well as washing your hair will help wash away radioactive perspiration. If you prepare food for others, wear rubber gloves to prevent your perspiration from getting in their food.

The Rules to Live by for 10 Days

- Minimize contact with small children or pregnant women.
- Use separate towels and sheets; wash separately.
- Wash your clothes and underwear separately.
- Flush toilet two or three times after use.
- Pee like a woman if you're a man.
- Do not share your bodily fluids.

If you're nursing, and are newly diagnosed with thyroid cancer, or require a follow-up scan, discuss delaying RAI treatment until you wean (in some cases it won't make a difference). *Otherwise, you must stop nursing and wean.* For more information on weaning, consult *The Breastfeeding Sourcebook*, 3rd edition.

7

THE IMPORTANCE OF FOLLOW-UP SCANS, TREATMENTS, AND BLOOD TESTS

If you've had papillary or follicular thyroid cancer in any stage, you'll be offered a whole body scan after a thyroidectomy to check for remnants of thyroid and thyroid cancer cells throughout your body, and to determine whether you need radioactive iodine therapy as a treatment (see previous chapter). There's also a blood test known as the thyroglobulin test (Tg test), which is used to detect whether there are any remaining thyroid cancer cells; this blood test only works if you've had a total thyroidectomy and RAI treatment, and is even more sensitive if you're prepared to go off your thyroid hormone medication or are injected with artificial TSH (Thyrogen®). If thyroglobulin is detectable, it's a sign of recurrence. If you had medullary thyroid cancer, you'd have, instead, a blood test that checks for calcitonin, which is the hormone made by the medullary cancer cells (see chapter 4). If your type of thyroid cancer lost (or never had) the ability to take up RAI, then other nuclear scans (thallium, Sestamibi, PET) and radiological studies (X-rays, CT scans, MRI scans) will be used to look for signs of thyroid cancer.

Once you have "clean" scans as well as undetectable levels of thyroglobulin in your blood, and clean radiology tests (CT scans, MRI scans, or X-rays) and there's no evidence of thyroid cancer left, you'll be put on life-long thyroid hormone. People with papillary or follicular cancers will be put on a "suppression dosage" to keep the TSH level at 0.1 mIU/L or less, while those with medullary thyroid cancers will take a "replacement dosage" to keep the TSH in its normal range.

This chapter discusses what's involved in preparing for the various scans and follow-up treatments for thyroid cancer.

Preparing for the Whole Body Scans (WBS)

The point of the whole body scan is to check for evidence of thyroid cancer cells throughout your body. But since you're taking your thyroid replacement hormone to maintain your thyroid hormone levels so you aren't hypothyroid, you'll be suppressing a valuable hormone that "wakes up" these cells so they can be found. That hormone is thyroid stimulating hormone or TSH. TSH makes thyroid cells "grow," produce thyroglobulin (a unique protein which marks the presence of these cancer cells), and suck up iodine, permitting radioactive iodine to identify and kill these cells. That way, if there are any left in your body after initial thyroid cancer treatment, you'll want to be able to detect them and treat them, relying upon an increased TSH level to cause the cells to suck up the radioactive iodine for a scan or treatment. Typically, whole body scans involve going off thyroid hormone for four to six weeks to deliberately induce a hypothyroid state, causing your TSH levels to increase to more than 30 mIU/L, which would "stimulate" any thyroid cancer cells left to "stand and be counted." This is known as the "withdrawal scan." The same thing is also done when you're finally given radioactive iodine (RAI) as a treatment for thyroid cancer.

Conventional "Withdrawal Scans"

"Withdrawal scans" are planned at least six weeks in advance. This is because it takes this length of time for the thyroid hormone levels to be totally depleted. The first four weeks are made tolerable by taking a short-acting form of thyroid hormone (liothyronine), Cytomel®, twice daily. In the final two weeks, the low iodine diet is started (see the next section) and you're advised to avoid driving or similar skilled activities because you're quite slow and tired. A small radioactive iodine "scan dose" is then given and a nuclear scan performed from one to three days later. Should the scan show residual thyroid tissue or evidence of thyroid cancer anywhere in your body, you're already prepared to be treated with a treatment dose of radioactive iodine. Although it's uncomfortable to be hypothyroid since all bodily functions are slowed down, the radioactive iodine persists long enough in the body to be taken up by any thyroid cancer cells. Following this, you resume your usual thyroid hormone dose and diet.

Thyrogen Scans

Now there's an alternative way of doing a thyroid scan after a thyroidectomy for patients who are considered likely to be free of residual cancer. This method is used for follow-up assessments after conventional "withdrawal scans" have been negative for evidence of cancer, and it's far more comfortable for you. A product known as Thyrogen® uses recombinant DNA technology to make a synthetic thyroid stimulating hormone (TSH) to substitute for the natural TSH produced by withdrawal of thyroid hormone. This is used for thyroid cancer patients, who have been previously shown to be free of disease, to prepare for RAI scans to check for thyroid cancer recurrence. Basically, it's the same as natural TSH, allowing you to remain at normal thyroid hormone levels for your scan. Because bodily processes, particularly kidney function, are maintained in a normal state, the radioactive iodine is rapidly excreted. For this reason, the Food and Drug Administration (FDA) recommends that the radioiodine tracer dose be at least four millicuries, and that the time taken for each scan picture be at least 30 minutes.

Many nuclear medicine departments, which perform these scans, don't realize how important it is to spend this prolonged time for the scan pictures. Measurement of the thyroglobulin level at the time of the scan increases the sensitivity of the testing for the presence of thyroid cancer. This makes Thyrogen® most appropriate for people with low risk cancers and previously clean "withdrawal scans." In addition, Thyrogen is not approved for use during radioactive iodine therapies because it's possible that it may result in a less effective therapy as compared to one given with thyroid hormone withdrawal. On the other hand, if Thyrogen is appropriate for you, you can maintain a better quality of life and comfort as you prepare for follow-up radioiodine scans. And while the hypothyroid preparation method often prevents people from working or driving while off of thyroid hormone, Thyrogen permits them to continue in their occupations and normal lifestyle while undergoing testing for their thyroid cancer.

Thyroglobulin Testing

Thyroglobulin is a protein, which is only made by thyroid cells or thyroid cancer cells. No other part of the body can make this special protein. Usually, thyroid or thyroid cancer cells release this protein into the blood, making it possible to measure it in a blood sample. Since there is no other source of thyroglobulin, once the thyroid gland has been completely removed by surgery and its remnants destroyed by radioactive iodine, there should be no measurable thyroglobulin left in the blood. Under these conditions, the presence of measurable thyroglobulin indicates the presence of thyroid cancer. It's important not to confuse the thyroglobulin level with the thyroglobulin antibody level or a thyroxine binding globulin level, which are both unrelated and often confused by patients and doctors for the thyroglobulin level.

You should be having a blood test for thyroglobulin at least every six months. This will only be an accurate indicator of a thyroid cancer recurrence if you've had a total thyroidectomy followed by radioactive iodine therapy. The thyroglobulin test is more accurate when TSH is not suppressed; the usual method is to perform Tg tests while hypothyroid or with Thyrogen®, when appropriate. Some physicians believe that selected patients with low risks of thyroid cancer recurrence may be evaluated with Thyrogen®-stimulated Tg testing once their scans are clean, and they're having regular thyroglobulin tests with results that are so low as to be undetectable. It's important to account for cancers that may have lost the ability to make Tg or take up RAI. This can be assessed with additional imaging tests (such as MRI scans or CT scans without contrast dye), as well as nuclear scans using radioactive thallium, MIBI, or radioactive sugar (PET scan).

Around one quarter or more of thyroid cancer patients (particularly women) have immune systems that produce antibodies against their own thyroglobulin. The reasons for this are not clearly understood and they do not directly influence your health; however they can make thyroglobulin testing difficult or impossible. This is because these antibodies interfere with the blood test for thyroglobulin performed in the laboratory, and prevent the thyroglobulin level in your blood from being accurately measured. For this reason, it is standard practice to measure both the thyroglobulin level and the thyroglobulin antibody level each time a thyroglobulin assessment is made. If the thyroglobulin antibody level is undetectable, then the measured thyroglobulin level may be considered reliable. If thyroglobulin antibody level is above the normal values for the laboratory, then you cannot rely upon the thyroglobulin level to see if you have persistent thyroid cancer.

Scanning is stressful and is not an insignificant burden on your physical and mental health. If you are in good health and have responded well to treatment, it's important that the interval scans be long enough to reflect the lack of evidence of cancer. On the other hand, if there's evidence of persistent cancer, it's important that appropriate treatments be applied if available. There's no value in performing scans that show the presence of thyroid cancer without treating the cancer. Likewise, if all evidence suggests the absence of this cancer, frequent scans are unnecessary and possibly bad for your health. Some doctors with experience in treating thyroid cancer increase the time interval between clean scans, with undetectable thyroglobulin levels, by one year as each scan is shown to be clean. In the near future, there may be a much more sensitive test, known as (it's a mouthful) the "quantitative reverse-transcriptase-polymerase chain reaction for thyroglobulin mRNA" in circulating blood or the "q-RT-PCR." This test may permit your doctor to actually measure the presence of thyroid cancer cells in your blood, unaffected by antibodies to thyroglobulin. Right now, this test is being evaluated in research studies to see if it's accurate enough to be developed for future clinical use.

How does thyroid hormone withdrawal or Thyrogen work?

By going off your thyroid hormone, your TSH levels rise, which can awaken thyroid cancer cells that have been "hibernating" since they were deprived of the TSH that's suppressed by the higher thyroid hormone dosages used in "suppression" therapy. This allows hidden, persistent thyroid cancer cells to be detected by either a scan or a thyroglobulin (Tg) test. Elevated TSH levels cause any thyroid cancer cells that might still be lurking around to do one (or both) of two things: make thyroglobulin, releasing it into your bloodstream (which is why a thyroglobulin blood test is so important—what a "Tg test" stands for on your medical records); and/or absorb radioactive iodine (which is what permits the cancer to be seen on the body scan). By taking synthetic TSH (Thyrogen®) you can create similar testing conditions without going off your thyroid hormone. But there are other issues surrounding this, discussed further on.

Is taking Thyrogen the best method?

Temporarily stopping your thyroid hormone and naturally forcing your own TSH levels up makes a scan or Tg test the most sensitive it can be and, indeed, many doctors advise against Thyrogen® for this reason; their philosophy is that they don't want to risk missing a thyroid cancer recurrence or underestimating the extent of the disease. But since the sensitivity in testing is not as critical in some people with very low risks of having left-over tumor, many doctors feel that quality of life is a more important benefit of the test using Thyrogen®. You see, the downside of being temporarily off of your thyroid hormone medication is that you may not feel well at all because you'll be hypothyroid: sluggish, tired, depressed, constipated, bloated, and the rest of the hypoalphabet soup of symptoms. Walk around that way for a month, and your quality of life can be seriously diminished. Given a choice, a lot of patients would rather trade general well being for a difference in scan or Tg test accuracy. Thyrogen is therefore a potential option for you if:

- You adamantly refuse to walk around hypothyroid prior to your scan.

- You don't need a scan, but do need a thyroglobulin test—yet want it to be more accurate than it would normally be unless TSH was there to stimulate it.

- You need to have a scan, and are willing to walk around hypothyroid, but you have other health problems that will be worsened by your hypothyroidism, such as severe depression, emotional disturbances, or neurological problems.

- You've had pituitary or hypothalamic (brain) disease, which prevents your body from making its own TSH.

- You and your physician are confident that there's a low chance that you'll need RAI treatment (since such treatment may not be as effective when using Thyrogen®).

Thyrogen® is not recommended if:

- You want the MOST accurate scan (and thyroglobulin blood test) possible, and don't want to risk a cancer being missed.

- You've only had a partial thyroidectomy; in this case you cannot get any RAI scanning using any method, since the entire thyroid must be surgically removed before RAI can be used.

• You're known to have recurrent or persistent thyroid cancer and will need to get RAI treatment.

• You're pregnant or nursing (the drug hasn't been tested on pregnant or nursing women and is therefore contraindicated). In this case, you should also avoid any radioactive scans or therapies.

• You have not previously had a "clean" RAI "withdrawal scan" with an undetectable Tg level.

• You're known to have a particularly aggressive type of thyroid cancer or tumor spread outside of the neck region.

• You don't have sufficient health care insurance coverage or you have limited finances (the injections cost over $1,000 US and over $1,500 Canadian).

How do you take Thyrogen®?

Thyrogen® is taken as an intramuscular injection given to you by your healthcare provider, and can literally be a "pain in the ass" because you have the injections in your buttocks area (or arm), and have to start the injections a few days before your test (you'll require two or three, depending on the circumstances). If you're having a scan, you'll take your radioactive iodine tracer the day after your last Thyrogen® injection, and will have your scan two days following the radioiodine dose.

Low Iodine Diet (LID)

Planning to go out for a lobster dinner the night before your whole body scan or radioactive iodine treatment? Don't bet on it. It's now standard practice to go on a low iodine diet two weeks before your scan. This involves avoiding certain medicines and foods that contain iodine for two weeks before your scan for more accurate results and greater effectiveness of RAI therapy. And since certain diagnostic procedures involve the use of iodine (particularly all intravenous contrast dyes used for CT scans and angiograms), be sure to let your doctor know what diagnostic procedures you've had. In general, a low iodine diet consists of very fresh foods prepared from fresh meats, fresh poultry, fresh or frozen vegetables, and fresh fruits. You are not permitted to use any dairy products, egg yolks, iodized salt, or Red Food Dye #3. While you're at it, you may even slim down, if you need to lose weight. That said, low iodine diets can be simple to follow and are a very small price to pay to ensure the greatest benefit from RAI scans and therapy.

In my day and region, there was no recommendation of a LID; today, we know that the less non-radioactive iodine in your body prior to taking RAI as a tracer or treatment, the less it will interfere with the uptake of the RAI. People make the mistake of assuming iodine means sodium because of iodized salt. A low iodine diet isn't the same thing as a low sodium diet. You can have salt as long as it isn't iodized salt. While most canned goods containing salt are not made with iodized salt, there's no reliable way to know which type has been added, and it'is safest to get foods without salt, adding your own non-iodized salt. Iodized salt, sea salt and salted foods are the things to avoid. Non-iodized salt (such as Kosher salt or salt labeled as without iodine) may be used. You may also want to avoid dining out if you want to stick to your LID.

For people who may not have access to fresh foods, which include people with low-incomes or people who live in remote areas, it's important to note that a LID doesn't have to be expensive; avoiding fast foods and prepared foods and substituting for simple fresh foods is healthier and cheaper. See the Appendix for a wonderful low iodine cookbook, reprinted from The Light of Life Foundation, a thyroid cancer organization.

Sources of iodine include:

(listed alphabetically)

- Chocolate (for its milk content).

- Commercial bakery products. It's not hard to bake your own delicious bread using: unbleached flour, sugar or honey, yeast, non-iodized salt, and olive oil.

- Cured and corned foods (ham, corned beef, sauerkraut, bacon, sausage, salami)—unless you produce your own using non-iodized salt.

- Dairy: milk, butter, cream, cheese (these products provide us with a large amount of our iodine). The iodine gets into dairy because the animals secret dietary iodine into their milk, while cows' teats are washed in iodine. Also, commercial milking machines are often washed with iodine cleansers.

- Eggs (whites are fine).

- Fish or seafood (this includes both fresh and saltwater fish).

- Food additives: carrageen, agar-agar, algin, alginate.

- Molasses.

- Sea salt or iodized salt (found in potato chips, popcorn, nuts, pretzels, restaurant foods). Keep in mind that kosher salt or non-iodized salt is fine, and sodium in any form is fine so long as it's not iodized salt.

- Seaweed or kelp (this is loaded with iodine!).

- Soy products (soy sauce, soymilk, tofu).

- Vitamins and supplements. Many of these contain iodine; check labels. Any red, orange or brown pills and capsules may have iodine dyes in them. (Ask your pharmacist to check: only Red Dye #3 needs to be avoided.)

RAI Treatment Decisions

If your first whole body scan showed remnants of thyroid tissue or spread of your cancer to other parts of your body, having the full RAI treatment will be recommended. As discussed in chapter 6, initial radioactive iodine treatment for most thyroid cancer involves a moderate dosage that ranges between 100 and 150 millicuries. This dosage is usually reserved for papillary and follicular cancers as well as Hurthle cell cancers, although it may not be that effective. For some types of thyroid cancers, particularly those that have invaded into areas of the neck outside of the thyroid gland or have spread to other parts of the body, the radioactive iodine dose may be much higher. After a therapeutic dose of radioactive iodine (i.e., over 100 millicuries), you're kept in isolation in a private hospital room for one to two days, and are not permitted any visitors. Chapter 6 outlines radioactive iodine side effects (there are very few), as well as the post-treatment precautions. All experts agree that when all normal thyroid tissue is destroyed with RAI therapy, it's a lot easier to use the blood test measuring levels of thyroglobulin (a protein made by thyroid tissue, discussed previously), to reveal residual or recurrent thyroid carcinoma. If you're making thyroglobulin that can be measured in your blood after your thyroid gland has been removed, and all the leftover bits (called "remnant tissue") destroyed, it's a sign that your cancer is still present.

Prior to RAI treatment, you'll need to be off your thyroid hormone and in a hypothyroid state. Thyrogen® is not recommended for RAI treatment; it's only recommended for follow-up scanning.

Treat and Repeat

Six months after your RAI treatment, you'll undergo another whole body scan. The testing strategy can differ dramatically from physician to physician and from place to place. In a typical approach, if you have a clean scan (and both undetectable Tg level and no evidence of tumor by other radiological procedures), you'll just be followed with another scan (each time checking Tg) in one year, then another in two years, and yet another in three years. Each time the interval between negative scans extends another year until a five-year interval is reached, and this interval is repeated indefinitely. Some physicians suggest substituting a hypothyroid (or Thyrogen®-stimulated Tg assessment) for some or all of these later scans. Such an approach is controversial. This is because not every thyroid cancer is able to produce Tg, and more than one-quarter of people make antibodies in their blood that make the Tg test untrustworthy. It's important for you to have confidence that your physician has considered these issues, and has individualized the method of monitoring your cancer. Any time a scan shows recurrent cancer, further RAI treatment is advised, usually at higher dosages than given previously. And if tumor is discovered outside of the neck region, it's often appropriate to give very high RAI doses, often exceeding 200 millicuries. Administration of such high doses requires distinct expertise (which could necessitate traveling to specialized centers), and techniques of "dosimetry" that permit the physician to calculate the highest RAI dose that can be given safely. If tumor is discovered by Tg tests, but does not take up RAI on scanning, it's often treated with surgery and external beam radiation therapy.

External Radiation

If you've had a thyroidectomy with the surrounding lymph nodes removed, and under a microscope your cancer appears to be a particularly aggressive type that won't respond to RAI, your surgeon may want you to have radiotherapy, or external radiation therapy. Sometimes it's recommended regardless of a clean scan following RAI therapy if persistent cancer, which doesn't respond to RAI, is discovered. Usually the purpose of external radiation therapy is to kill thyroid cancer cells that are too small to find and remove surgically, when there's no other way to more effectively deliver the radiation. If the RAI is sufficiently effective, nearly five times more radiation might be able to be delivered to each cancer cell; however external radiation therapy is used when RAI is not an option.

Radiation therapy (XRT) involves a type of X-ray beam treatment. It's often confused with chemotherapy (see chapter 5). Your hair will not fall out, nor will you experience any nausea, or any other side effects associated with chemotherapy. On the other hand, XRT causes mild to severe irritation of the esophagus, which lasts from several weeks to months. This may result in decreased food intake, as it can be very difficult to swallow. Sometimes the neck also gets quite stiff and the skin looks as if it's been severely sunburned. Regular stretching exercises, time and patience should restore you to your normal state, but it could take over a year. Attentive care by your radiation oncologist (the type of doctor who arranges and manages XRT) should get you over the rough times.

The actual process of preparing for XRT, however, is a little complex. First, you'll be referred to the radiation oncologist, who is not the same doctor coordinating RAI therapy (that would be a nuclear medicine specialist). The radiation oncologist will "tattoo" you by injecting a tiny dot of special dye in a precise area of your neck. This dot will look like a small, blue freckle, and will ensure that the aim of the X-ray beam is on target each day of therapy.

A total dose of radiation is then determined, which is subsequently fractionated into smaller weekly doses the way an annual salary is broken up into weekly pay. A few days after you're tattooed, you'll report to a radiation clinic, located in the hospital basement. Radiation clinics are situated in the basement because hospitals want to minimize the risk of radiation exposure to healthy people. It's really a just a convenient way to assist in shielding the equipment; however, reporting to a clinic in the bowels of a hospital feels very isolating and depressing. That's why it's important to bring someone along for support, so make sure you don't go alone.

The radiation clinic will have a number of radiotechnicians on staff who will operate the actual machinery. The equipment can vary from hospital to hospital. Although the procedure itself is painless, the after-effects are not. Knowing this in advance may not alleviate the symptoms, but it may make them more understandable, and therefore more bearable. External radiation kills the cells inside by causing damage to their DNA (genes). By week two, the squared-off area that the beam targets will look like a very bad sunburn, and your throat will feel extremely sore. Swallowing will be very painful. As the treatment progresses, your throat will become tender. You'll also feel quite tired by the third or fourth week of treatment, because the procedure is mentally as well as physically draining.

To help with the sunburn symptoms, avoid soaps or lotions with perfume in them, and request a consult with a dermatologist who can recommend the right cream to soothe the burn. Lavender oil is reportedly helpful for burns as well. Obviously, eating soft foods will be better. Or, if you're turned off food altogether, you could survive on liquid meal supplement. As soon as the treatments are finished, you'll start to feel much better. This is usually followed up with another CAT scan in about three months.

You must be vigilant about wearing sunscreen to protect your treated area. Both the American and Canadian cancer societies publish these "SunSense" guidelines:

1. Reduce sun exposure between 11am and 4pm, when the sun's rays are the strongest. If you can, plan your outdoor activities before or after this time. It's easy to remember this time—during these hours your shadow is shorter than you are!

2. Seek shade or create your own shade. When you're outside, especially between 11am and 4pm, try to stay in the shade. Be prepared for places without any shade by taking along an umbrella. With an umbrella you can create shade wherever you need it.

3. Slip! On clothing to cover your arms and legs. Covering your skin will protect it from the sun. Choose clothing that's loose fitting, tightly woven, lightweight.

4. Slap! On a wide-brimmed hat. Most skin cancers occur on the face and neck, so this area needs extra protection. Wear a hat with a wide brim that covers your head, face, ears and neck. Hats without a wide brim, like baseball caps, do not give you enough protection.

5. Slop! On a sunscreen with a Sun Protection Factor (SPF) of #15 or higher. Look for "broad spectrum" on the label. This means that the sunscreen offers protection against two types of ultraviolet rays, UV-A and UV-B. Apply sunscreen generously, 20 minutes before outdoor activities. Reapply frequently, at least every two hours, and after swimming or exercise that makes you perspire. Remember that no sunscreen can absorb all of the sun's rays. Use sunscreen along with shade, clothing and hats, not instead of them. Use sunscreen as a back up in your sun protection plan.

Thyroid Hormone Suppression Therapy

If you've had papillary or follicular thyroid cancer, you'll be placed on what's called a suppression dosage of thyroid hormone. Any microscopic bit of thyroid cancer in your body may be stimulated by TSH–meaning that the TSH may stimulate cancerous tissue to grow. In your case, the trick is to find a high enough dosage to suppress your TSH (which means that blood tests will show that you have higher free T4 readings than hypothyroid patients who are merely taking thyroid hormone to keep themselves in the normal range). TSH suppression can be accomplished without causing you to become hyperthyroid (where you have too much thyroid hormone), using precise daily doses with brand name thyroid hormone (levothyroxine) pills. It's critical to take the pill every morning, and to make up doses missed by taking them as soon as remembered, even if it requires more than one pill to be taken at once. The pills are very sensitive to heat and will become easily inactive when exposed to temperatures warm enough to soften a chocolate bar. The average dose needed for TSH suppression is roughly two micrograms for every kilogram of body weight; but this can vary.

One study found that patients on thyroid hormone specifically for TSH suppression were better off waiting one hour after taking their pill in the morning before having breakfast. Certain medications, such as iron supplements or vitamins that contain iron, will block the absorption of thyroid hormone if taken within five hours of taking the thyroid hormone tablet. In addition, it's important to learn what your thyroid hormone tablets look like so that you can be safe from pharmacist errors. For full information on thyroid hormone replacement, including T3, brands, dosing by weight, contraindications and side effects (including signs of hyperthyroidism), please consult *The Thyroid Sourcebook, 4th Edition* or *The Hypothyroid Sourcebook*.

The TSH test will determine whether your TSH levels are being suppressed enough, and whether you are hypo- or hyperthyroid (from too little or too much). The TSH level should be less than or equal to 0.1 mIU/L. Most general physicians will try to reduce your thyroid hormone dosage, not realizing that the normal TSH values for hypothyroid patients without cancer are not applicable to thyroid cancer patients. For this reason, it's important make sure that you know your TSH levels and make sure that the physician is properly informed.

Treating Recurrence

Recurrence of papillary or follicular thyroid cancer often means a similar round of RAI scans and treatments all over again, perhaps further surgery, and possibly external beam radiation therapy. Sometimes there's a distant spread of papillary or follicular cancer to other organs. If this is the case, you may be offered dosimetry-directed RAI therapy or, if there's no RAI uptake, the opportunity to participate in experimental clinical trials using new chemotherapy agents (see chapter 5). Recurrence for Hurthle cell or medullary thyroid cancers may involve such experimental chemotherapy as well, or external beam radiation therapy. Anaplastic cancer is a final stage of a typically fatal thyroid cancer, which is unresponsive to most known therapies, and so recurrence, in this case, is not a relevant topic (see chapter 5).

8

EMOTIONAL, PSYCHOLOGICAL, AND SPIRITUAL ISSUES

As a thyroid cancer survivor myself, I've spent years feeling "outside the box" in terms of finding support from cancer organizations. People who've gone through thyroid cancer don't experience the same treatments as many other cancer patients. The combination of having a very treatable cancer as well as radioactive iodine therapy makes us unique. The fact that most of us do not undergo chemotherapy is also unique. But we're then cast into the "pool" of thyroid disease sufferers, the majority of whom have been diagnosed with *primary* hypo- or hyperthyroidism. But we have secondary hypothyroidism, caused by the treatment for our cancer, and must be on thyroid hormone replacement for life. Among other thyroid sufferers we're "unique" and among other cancer patients we're "unique." Alone, isolated, and without other people who've gone through what we have, many of us thyroid cancer patients feel as though we're the only ones we know of with this sort of cancer. Well, those days are over! There are several sources of support for thyroid cancer survivors. Please consult the Resources at the back of the book.

When planning the content for this book, every thyroid cancer survivor I spoke to made a special point of discussing the psychosocial aspects of thyroid cancer, and how they're typically ignored in most materials. This chapter is designed to address the emotional aspects of having thyroid cancer, which can include coping with fatigue, depression, anxiety, and panic. Thyroid cancer also affects friends and family members, and can change communication patterns and relationships. Finally, our spirits and souls need nourishment. Cancer has cut through our belief systems, and has made us aware of our mortality. Some of us change or question our beliefs; some of us make significant changes in our lives and relationships as a result of cancer. Cancer can set us off on a journey of self-discovery, a journey that's triggered by the awareness of our mortality. So this chapter includes material from the philosophical and spiritual literature—in consultation with clergy—on suffering, mortality, and passion. These are topics I have dealt with extensively in other works.

The Passion of Cancer

The Greek word, "passio" means suffering; it's also the root word of "passion." Most people define passion as happiness, joy, and sexual fulfillment. But passion really just means "feeling your life." Feeling the essence of life: real feelings, real suffering, and raw emotions. Having cancer is a passionate act. When we go through it, we're living on a sort of "edge" or "cliff" waiting for the unknown, and calling on *all* our inner reserves and strength to get through the experience.

Feeling Our Mortality

When we feel our lives, we're feeling our mortality. As we age, we become particularly aware of our mortality—especially when illness or loss strikes. When we experience illness, and/or physical vulnerability, our lives take on new meaning, and we begin to look at them differently. Gail Sheehy, author of *Passages*, refers to this as the "task of reflection." It's often upon this reflection (did we "live well," are we happy, were we good people, are there things we still want, or need to do…etc.), that we become more passionate, but this usually results when we make a conscious shift to another stage of life. At this stage in life, our health, for example, suddenly becomes very important to us; many people become active for the first time, or dramatically change their lifestyle habits—eating well, quitting smoking, and so on.

Feeling our mortality may sound ominous, but if you didn't know you were going to die one day, you wouldn't find enjoyment in anything you did. There would be no "last piece of cake," sense of time, sense of something being "over." Nor would there be that "last night" on a vacation. Without these small, daily reminders that we won't last forever, our lives would, in fact, be devoid of meaning. At the same time, without endings there'd be no beginnings. There'd be nothing "new," such as a new food to explore, new places to go, new people to meet, and so on. Without a sense of the "new" there'd be no value in art or the artist, as it's the uniqueness and "newness" of an artist's work that we appreciate and place value in. Without feeling our deaths, we can't feel our lives, you see.

I've thought about this a lot because of my own cancer experience. In my own life, I've often been "scolded" by friends and loved ones for working too much or too hard. I'm told that I'm a workaholic, when, in fact, I feel this is an untrue statement. But when I explored the reasons why I produce at the rate that I do, I realized it had to do with "feeling" my mortality. Because I had thyroid cancer at an early age, and have faced the prospect of my own death, I have a sense of urgency about my work. If I knew I'd live forever, I wouldn't be concerned with my deadlines, productivity, and so forth. So "the meaning of life" is the meaning of death. Without death, there'd be no meaning to our lives; but without a meaningful life, our deaths would have no meaning, either. It's a difficult Catch 22. Thus, passion is the act of feeling our lives by appreciating our future, and eventual death. The character, Morrie, in *Tuesdays with Morrie* states: "when you know how to die, you know how to live."

Suffering

First of all, we suffer because we're aware. And the more awareness we have about our lives, the more we can suffer. All human beings suffer; it's part of what it means to be human and to grow. But there are different kinds of suffering human beings endure and, more specifically, different kinds of suffering *we* endure that may not lead to growth but instead to a diminished quality of life. Physical pain, for example, can trigger suffering that doesn't necessarily lead to emotional growth.

Suffering can develop when we realize our lives or situations are not improving, or are even declining. Stagnating, or "being in a rut," or finding our lives are getting worse, rather than better, are conditions that lead to suffering. As human beings, once our basic needs (safety, food, shelter, love) are looked after, we're driven toward self-actualization. But when our life circumstances stymie self-actualization or spiritual growth, we suffer. The longing for material possessions, money or an intimate relationship is often just an expression of longing for self-realization. Later in life, many of us also begin to question our attachments to material possessions and power, and, as we get older, begin to see the difference between real needs (i.e., love, friendship, respect) and artificial needs (i.e., money, power, or prestige).

For those of us who like the status quo and the quality of life we've already attained, suffering can develop when a life event of some kind threatens that—jeopordizing our identity or self-hood. The "threat" can come from an infinite variety of sources, including illness.

Indeed, suffering can have a positive outcome. In other words, no pain, no gain! When you're in a rut, or feel trapped by life's circumstances, the suffering you feel can be your mind's and body's way of saying *wake up and change*! In this case, the only way to *stop* the suffering, would be to change the conditions of your life (as in leaving a stagnant marriage) or, at least, change the way you *view* the conditions of your life (as in "my infertility isn't a curse after all—it's actually allowed me to go back to school and change professions). In other words, if you can't change your life, you can still change your *perspective* on it, which can be a huge life-changing event, even though the circumstances remain the same.

When it's your body that's triggering your suffering (as in a physical illness), the process of disease and illness can lead to a new and evolved perspective on life. On an emotional level, growth has been compared to peeling an onion; *the more you peel, the more you cry*. Confronting fears, looking at painful memories, and so forth are all experiences that trigger emotional growth and maturity.

Suffering that doesn't lead to personal growth or illumination (which often occurs in the face of mortality, aging, terminal illness, etc.) is probably a good definition of "hell." Why suffer unless something better will result from it? Indeed, suffering may not yield immediate tangible results. An interesting concept is one that Talmudic scholars call the "hiding face of God"—an argument used to deal with the problem of evil. (If a good, kind God exists, why is there so much evil in the world?) The argument goes something like this: since the life span of one human being is so short compared to the life span of the human race (or God), it's not always possible to understand *why* God "hides its face" when individual humans appear to be suffering needlessly; there may be a good reason for our suffering, but we won't live long enough to understand the outcome. For example, a mouse used in cancer research would be suffering without the knowledge that its suffering is contributing to a cancer cure, which could potentially prevent the suffering of millions of people in the future.

Many people appear to suffer for no good reason. But if you're aware that you're suffering, you are, in fact, living a passionate existence. If you can learn something new, feel something new or change direction as a result of your suffering, you're growing. And this is an indication that you're alive, and part of the human race—it means you're feeling your life—something passionate people do.

Feeling Connected

The large body of work that looks at causes of suffering, sadness, and depression shows us that people suffer most when they're feeling out of connection with the world around them. When we feel "plugged in" to our community and network of friends and colleagues, it brings us increased zest, well-being, and motivation. *That's why connecting with other thyroid cancer survivors is so important.* Connection brings us increased self-worth, as well as a desire to make more connections.

Often, cancer makes us want to cocoon, and isolate ourselves even more. But cutting ourselves off from people can also cause loneliness. Loneliness is stressful; solitude is rejuvenating. Loneliness comes from a lack of truly intimate relationships with friends or family members; intimacy, in this case, refers to sharing deep feelings, fears and so on with someone else. This is how we unburden ourselves and relieve stress. Feeling as though you belong somewhere, or feeling part of a community can also alleviate loneliness. If you don't have support from your family, try to connect with other thyroid cancer survivors. See the back of this book for resources.

Coping with Depression

In the majority of cases, people suffering from depression have *unipolar depression*, a mood disorder characterized by one low mood. This is distinct from *bipolar depression*, a mood disorder in which there are two moods: one high mood and one low mood. This book will show you ways to modify your lifestyle and reduce stress, which may prevent the development of a unipolar depression; it doesn't discuss bipolar depression.

Most cases of unipolar depression are caused by life circumstances and/or situations. For this reason, the term "situational depression" is used by mental health care experts to describe most cases of mild, moderate or even severe unipolar depression. Situational depression can first mean that your depression has been triggered by a life event. Examples of a "life event" include:

- illness;
- loss of a loved one (the relationship may have ended, or a loved one may have died);
- major life change;
- job loss or change; or
- moving.

Depression is distinct from sadness in that it's a point *beyond* it, characterized by a numbness and inability to act. Depression is clinically known as a "mood disorder." It's impossible to define what a "normal" mood is since we all have such complex personalities, and exhibit different moods throughout a given week, or even a given day. But it's not impossible for *you* to define what a "normal" mood is for *you*. You know how you feel when you're functional: you're eating, sleeping, interacting with friends and family, being productive, active, and generally interested in the daily goings-on of life. Well, depression is when you feel you've *lost* the ability to function for a prolonged period of time or, if you're functioning at a reasonable level to the outside world, you've lost *interest* in participating in life.

One bad day, or even one bad week (which will usually include some "relief time" where you *can* laugh at something or take pleasure in something) from time to time is not a sign that you're depressed. Feeling you've lost the ability to function as you *normally* do all day, every day, for a period of at least two weeks, may be a sign that you're depressed. The symptoms of depression can vary from person to person, but can include some or all of the following:

- feelings of sadness and/or "empty mood;"
- difficulty sleeping (usually waking up frequently in the middle of the night);
- loss of energy and feelings of fatigue and lethargy;
- change in appetite (usually a loss of appetite);
- difficulty thinking, concentrating, or making decisions;
- loss of interest in formerly pleasurable activities, including sex;
- anxiety or panic attacks;
- obsessing over negative experiences or thoughts;
- feeling guilty, worthless, hopeless, or helpless;
- feeling restless and irritable; and
- thinking about death or suicide.

When You Can't Sleep

The typical sleep pattern of a depressed person is to go to bed at the normal time, only to wake up around 2 am, and find that getting back to sleep is impossible. Endless hours are spent watching infomercials to pass the time, or simply tossing and turning, usually obsessing over negative experiences or thoughts. Lack of sleep affects our ability to function, and leads to increased irritability, lack of energy and fatigue. Insomnia by itself is not a sign of depression, but when you look at depression as a package of symptoms, the inability to fall or stay asleep can aggravate all your other symptoms. In some cases, people who are depressed will oversleep, requiring 10 to 12 hours of sleep every night.

When You Can't Think Clearly

Another debilitating feature of depression is finding that you simply can't concentrate or think clearly. You feel scattered, disorganized, and unable to prioritize. This usually hits hardest in the workplace or at a center of learning, and can severely impair your performance. You may miss important deadlines, important meetings, or find you can't focus when you *do* go to meetings. When you can't think clearly, you can be overwhelmed with feelings of helplessness or hopelessness. "I can't even perform a simple task such as X anymore" may dominate your thoughts, while you become more and more frustrated with your dwindling productivity.

Anhedonia: When Nothing Gives You Pleasure

One of the most telling signs of depression is a loss of interest in activities that used to excite you, enthuse you, or give you pleasure. This is known as anhedonia, derived from the word "hedonism". You might tell your friends, for example, that you don't "have any desire" to do X or Y; you can't "get motivated;" or X or Y just doesn't "hold your interest or attention." You may also notice that your sense of satisfaction from a job well done is simply gone, which is particularly debilitating in the workplace or in a place of learning. For example, artists (photographers, painters, writers, etc.) may find that the passion has gone out of their work.

Many of the other symptoms of depression hinge on this "loss of pleasure," however. One of the reasons weight loss is so common in depression (typically, people may notice as much as a 10-pound drop in their weight) is because food no longer gives them pleasure, or cooking no longer gives them pleasure. The sense of satisfaction we get from having a clean home or clean kitchen may also disappear. Therefore, tackling cleaning up our kitchens in order to prepare food may be too taxing, contributing to a lack of interest in food.

Of course, many of you will be coping with hypothyroidism, which induces depression, too. In that case, consult my book *The Hypothyroid Sourcebook*.

Short-Term Treatment Strategies

There is no one way to "stop the suffering" in depression. Different things work for different people. Less invasive solutions involve finding someone to talk to. This translates into finding counseling or psychotherapy, which I discuss in chapter 9. Talk therapy may also work best in combination with antidepressants (which this book does not discuss) or self-healing strategies, discussed in chapter 9. The *"sharing"* approach has been shown to be highly beneficial—particularly in cases where people share difficult circumstances or have difficulties in common.

Finally, creativity is important when fighting depression. When people express their feelings through their work, art (by this, I mean art in all its forms: words, fine arts, visual arts, healing arts, performing arts, etc.), hobbies or sport, they're not only feeling their lives but *expressing their lives*. Creativity is an amazing defense against depression. Writing, in particular (in the form of journaling, poetry, or letter writing) is a great way to express yourself, and improve your mental health. A new study published in *The Journal of the American Medical Association* found that people suffering from chronic ailments such as asthma or arthritis actually felt better when they wrote about their ailments.

A few years ago, Oprah Winfrey used her influence to get her viewers to begin daily journaling or diary writing because of the powerful effects it can have on enabling those of us who are otherwise without voice or expression. Using *her* own creativity to enable others, she has "resold" the idea of journaling in an age where few people take the time to sit down and be still with their thoughts. Oprah has taken journaling one step further by encouraging people to begin "gratitude journaling" where they think about what, in their lives, they're thankful for, and actually write it down. A firm believer in literacy as well, Oprah's influence on the comeback of journals may also inspire and enable those of us who, in the past, were afraid to write because of education levels. For people who don't feel they're "creative" or "artistic," journaling is a way to express feelings and passions free of censure. Remember Megan Stendebach (see chapter 3)? She created *www.thyroidcancersongs.com*, and found humor to be a tremendous healing source for her thyroid cancer. The narrative I include in that same chapter is another great example of how one thyroid cancer survivor chose to cope.

Anxiety and Panic

When it comes to stress-related anxiety due to cancer, we're talking about something known as Generalized Anxiety Disorder (GAD). GAD is characterized by extreme worry about things that are unlikely to happen. You may worry about whether your child is safe, or whether your partner is going to get into a car accident on the way home. You may begin to worry about health problems in other family members or friends. The worries begin to be persistent, and interfere with your normal functioning. There's a sense of dread, a constant "fretting," restlessness and uneasiness about your personal security or safety. You may also suffer from physical symptoms:

- clenching teeth or jaw;
- tightened muscles;
- holding one's breath;
- sleeping problems;
- racing heart beat;
- breathing difficulties;
- chest pain; and
- hyperventilation.

It's normal to worry about a lot of things, especially when you're being treated for cancer. Worry crosses over into "anxiety" when the worry persists after the problem you worried about has resolved or ended. Normally, when a problem's been resolved, there's a calm or even a sense of satisfaction that follows. For example, if you were awaiting the results of a scan, you'd naturally worry and be anxious about it until you had the results. When the doctor tells you the scan is clean, it would be natural at this point to feel relief. When you suffer from anxiety, you don't get the relief. You begin to think…What if the doctor made a mistake? What if I'm not fine? This is anxiety. In other words, if you're always worrying about *something*, that worrying is a sign that you may benefit from counseling or therapy. Being in a constant state of worry disrupts your life and prevents you from functioning normally.

Health Anxiety

Cancer can create a distinct form of anxiety, known as health anxiety. This is when the anxiety/panic is confined to your health. People who suffer from health anxiety are usually healthy, but become overly sensitive to bodily sensations, and quickly jump from "what's this itch?" to the belief that their cancer has spread, or a new cancer has sprouted. People with health anxiety may go from doctor to doctor looking for "answers" to their symptoms, and become more and more frustrated when they're told that they're healthy, or that there's nothing wrong. Indeed, the symptoms of panic and anxiety resemble many physical symptoms that plague people with health anxiety, such as: numbness, tingling, stomach trouble, headaches, twitching, odd sensations, flushes, and heart palpitations. People with health anxiety may also spend hours on the Internet looking up rare diseases (what they're doing now has a name—cyberchondria), becoming convinced that they're dying from one thing on Monday, and another thing on Friday. They frequently have OCD, or obsessive compulsive disorder, where in these cases the obsessions are focused on the body. If you believe you suffer from health anxiety, a good website to visit is *www.healthanxiety.com*.

Panic Attacks

When you suffer from anxiety, you may also suffer from panic attacks. A panic attack is so named because it's an "attack"—it comes on suddenly without warning. Because there is no warning, once you've had one panic attack, you can easily begin to worry about when the next one will strike. The fear of reliving a panic attack in public can become so overwhelming you may be afraid to leave your home. This is known as agoraphobia: the fear of going outside. When you're home, you're in a safe place for a panic attack. But when you're in public, the panic is heightened, as can be the actual symptoms of the attack.

A rush of adrenaline—a stress hormone that gets pumped out in a "fight or flight" response, brings on the symptoms of a panic attack. People with diabetes who suffer from episodes of low blood sugar have the same response, as adrenaline gets pumped out when blood sugar is low. If you're suffering from anxiety, you often don't eat well, so panic attacks can be exacerbated by low blood sugar.

When the adrenaline pumps out, and the "fight or flight" response is triggered, you'll first feel an accelerated heart rate, which often feels not like a palpitation but a "fluttery" heart beat; it can also feel racing, pounding or skipping. This is accompanied by a cold sweat or excessive sweating, chills or flushes (a.k.a cold or hot flashes), and possibly tingling or numbness in parts of your body. What happens next depends on what's going on in your life. Some people begin to feel "vertigo" symptoms: extreme dizziness, lightheadedness, shakiness, and nausea and other stomach problems. Other people begin to feel "choking" symptoms: rapid breathing or hyperventilating, difficulty breathing, a choking or smothering sensation or a lump in the throat; chest pain, pressure, or discomfort.

As one therapist put it to me, people who feel their world is collapsing tend to have "vertigo-like" panic attacks as their symptoms mirror how they feel. Meanwhile, people who feel they have too much responsibility or weight on their shoulders, tend to have "choking-like" panic attacks, as their symptoms mirror how they feel, too.

Whether the symptoms are "vertigo" or "choking," there's also a feeling of unreality about panic attacks; you may feel you're in a nightmare or dream, or are detached from your body for the duration of the attack, with distorted perceptions. A fear of losing control or embarrassing yourself, sense of impending doom, or fear of dying may also be part of the experience. You may also pass out. When you begin to notice panic attack symptoms, you can start to panic even more because the situation is so frightening and jarring.

Roughly two percent of North Americans aged 18 to 54 suffer from panic attacks each year, and those attacks occur twice as often in women than men. Although chronic panic attacks often occur before age 24, many people suffer their first attacks in their 30s and 40s, while under extreme stress. This can trigger the part of the brain that controls the fear response. Stresses that can bring on panic attacks include all of the normal socio-economic problems I discussed above: relationship problems, health problems, job, or money problems.

Managing Anxiety and Panic

Talk therapy is an excellent way to manage anxiety and panic. Finding a good therapist can be challenging. See the section further on about finding good counseling. Although it's common for women to be tossed a prescription for antidepressants or tranquilizers by family doctors or psychiatrists, the research on treatment shows that talk therapy—particularly cognitive behavioral therapy (see further on)—is often the best way to manage anxiety and panic. When someone can validate what you're feeling and give you some real, hands-on life management skills as an anchor, it's amazing how much better you can feel. Antidepressants, anti-anxiety agents, and drugs that slow your heart down and calm you while in the throes of a panic attack have a role in treatment, too, but all reasonable mental health practitioners believe in *starting low, going slow*. You should always start with the least invasive therapy first, before you move on to something that could have side effects.

Next time you're in the throes of a panic attack, here are three natural things to try:

- Breathe into a paper bag. This will slow down your heart naturally, as you breathe in more carbon dioxide.
- Carry around "rescue remedy"—a homeopathic remedy for panic and anxiety that is part of the Bach line of flower remedies, available in natural pharmacies. These are drops you take orally when you feel the panic beginning.
- Carry the essential oil orange. This calms the heart. When you feel the panic coming on, apply the oil to the nape of your neck, the thymus gland at the front of your neck, and the soles of your feet. The oil should penetrate quickly and help calm you.

Coping with Fatigue

A typical day in the life of someone recovering from thyroid cancer surgery or RAI therapies and scans involves a collapse on the couch after a brief outing or errand. And this usually comes as quite a shock. In fact, many cancer patients list fatigue as one the most frustrating post-operative symptoms. That's why, even though you may feel fine at 7:00 in the morning, and feel like putting in a full day's work, you may want to give yourself some time to rest.

A common scenario is to plan a day's worth of activities and find that you can only accomplish one or two tasks before total exhaustion sets in. This fatigue is not caused so much by the surgery as it is by the events *surrounding* the surgery: stress, reorganization of lifestyle, decisions about post-surgical treatment, waiting for biopsy results, and dealing with concerned friends and family. Your body is also responding to recent changes in *its* environment—be it removal of axillary lymph nodes or removal of tissue.

The remedy for fatigue is obvious: REST! But finding the time to rest can be challenging. Here are some tips:

1. Forget "banking hours"—keep "toddler hours." Get up early and have a nice breakfast. (This is the best time to get things done!) Nap mid-morning. Nap after lunch. Have an early dinner, "bathtime" and go to bed by around 8:00 after reading a good story.

2. If you need to work for a living like most on the planet, try to arrange flex time so you can work early and get home early. You'll have much more energy in the early morning and poop out by early afternoon. You'll also avoid rush hour, which can tire anybody out. Or, try to build in time for a nap and go back to the office later.

3. Limit your errands. Shop and bank by phone; use more couriers to save yourself running back and forth; divide errands up between family members and friends.

4. Limit visitors and visiting only to places and people that give you *energy*. In other words, say "yes" to that "chick flick" with a good friend; "no" to that dysfunctional family brunch you promised your aunt you'd attend!

5. Next time someone asks, "Is there anything I can do?" ask the kind soul to run an errand you don't have the energy for!

6. Make a list of everything that needs to get done. Then cut it in half until only what *must* get done "today" gets done. Anything that can wait, *should*.

Eliminating Energy Drains

Coping with cancer is stressful; when I was ill, I spent more time reassuring others than taking time for myself to heal. Most energy drains come in the form of people. When people who take energy from you rather than give you energy in the form of support surround you, the result is more stress in your life. By doing a serious re-evaluation of your personal relationships, you may be able find more energy and reduce the amount of stress in your life. Ask yourself some of the following questions:

1. Do you have someone in your life that offers judgement-free emotional support? This means a person who makes you feel positive

about yourself rather than a person who points out your flaws or attacks your choices.

2. Are there people in your life who drain your energy and reserves? These are people who always seem to be in crisis, and suck up large amounts of "free therapy" time from you, but never seem to be there for you. These can also be people who criticize you and make you feel negative and hopeless instead of positive and optimistic.

3. Do you have unresolved conflicts with family members or friends? These unresolved feelings can drain your energy and focus as we tend to obsess over the conflict over and over again.

4. Do you feel your friends are more "acquaintances," and lack truly intimate friendships?

5. Is there someone in your life who continuously breaks commitments or plans, with whom you are constantly rescheduling?

Energy drains can also come from unmet needs in your home environment. Do you have broken appliances, car repairs that haven't been done, a wardrobe you hate, cluttered closets and rooms, or even ugly surroundings? Living in a home that's not decorated in a way that pleases you makes you feel as though you don't want to be there. Plants, paint, covers for ugly furniture, and a few things on the wall often make the difference between barren and dank surroundings and cozy. See chapter 9 about self-care for more on the "little things" in life that make huge differences to your stress quotient.

Finally, simply doing too much and expecting too much from ourselves drains our energy. Whenever possible, hire someone to do the things you can't or don't want to do. Consider hiring someone to:

- clean your house or apartment;
- de-clutter your house by going through closets, filing things, and so on;
- organize your tax receipts; or
- garden and/or take care of your lawn.

Cancer and Life Partners

Based on the literature surrounding psychosocial issues in cancer, most couples experience the "spousal scene." The ill partner goes into the appointment alone, while the well partner waits and experiences a "blackout" where no information about what's going on is being communicated. Meanwhile, the well partner may become more and more overwhelmed by the experience and less able to talk about it when s/he goes home. This sets up more difficult dynamics in the home, as one partner feels unable to fully participate in the experience. Many experts believe that a huge source of miscommunication occurs in this "blackout" period when one spouse is in the doctor's office and the other is waiting outside that office.

The first rule is to avoid these kinds of blackouts and make it clear to your team of doctors that you want your significant other to be *included* in all of your appointments. Thyroid cancer is complex, and requires, as discussed throughout this book, a series of decisions. Many of these decisions are lifestyle-centered, and will affect your spouse or partner and other family members. But a spouse or partner can play a much larger role than companionship in the appointment process. For example:

- Let your spouse listen with you in the appointment. There may be times when, as the patient, you feel too emotional and overwhelmed or too spacey to take in the amount of information that's thrown at you. Your spouse can help do the "listening" (although sometimes a spouse's anxiety can interfere with what s/he hears, too). In any event, two listeners are always better than one. Later, you can recap what went on and discuss the appointment in detail together.
- Let your partner/spouse help you by doing whatever s/he's good at, such as research, for example. If you're better at doing the research, fine; if s/he's better at it, let him or her handle that aspect. The important thing is that you both stay focused at helping each other. Many of the decisions you're faced with between appointments involve self-education. And that means doing Internet searches for more information; going to libraries or bookstores; or finding good support groups. If your spouse is good at "finger walking" and bringing home the informational "goodies," allow him or her to handle these tasks.
- Let your spouse ask the doctor questions, too. Your spouse may have questions you never thought to ask. This is a valuable contribution to the appointment. The more answers you get, the more equipped you are to make decisions.
- If possible, make the appointment day a pamper day, too. Often, doctor appointments take up a significant portion of the day. So *make* a day of it. Have a nice lunch before or after the appointment. Take in an afternoon movie. Get some "together" time in that doesn't revolve

around cancer. On the flip side, of course, many patients find the appointment day an anxious time. It brings up memories of the diagnosis and treatment. So acknowledge that you may feel worse than usual when this day rolls around, and allow yourself to have comfort, comfort foods, friends, and quiet support.

- Let your spouse take care of household details on "appointment day." Arranging for childcare or carpooling, small errands such as groceries, and so on.

If you're the well partner reading this, you'll want to know what strategies have worked for other spouses/partners dealing with cancer, and what it is that cancer patients *need* from their partners during this time. Consider the following:

- Become the homemaker without asking. Look after as many of the meals, chores and so on as you can. Sick people often have trouble asking for help and worry about how to get everything done. This automatically takes away the responsibility from the ill partner and makes it easier for her to rest without guilt.
- Random acts of romance. Whether it's impulsively taking a day off to go to the zoo; planning a romantic weekend away, or giving your spouse a rose for every appointment s/he made it through, these are small things that show caring and thought. It says: "I think about you when you're not around. I want to take you away from this. I want to be with you."
- Go to support groups. Whether it's a "just for spouses" support group or a couples group, go. This says: "I want to share the experience with you. I want to meet other people in the same situation so we can form meaningful friendships." One husband (whose wife had cancer) relayed that the most valuable experience he and his wife shared was a cancer support group held at their home. The husband had an opportunity to listen to the needs of all kinds of people with cancer, which ultimately helped bring him and his wife together.
- Random acts of research. Ask if anyone in your workplace has gone through thyroid cancer themselves, or with a spouse. Talk and share with others and bring home more information. Cut out meaningful articles and pick out books you think your partner would like. This says: "I think about you at work and throughout my day."
- Random acts of humor. You know your spouse better than anyone else. You know what would make him or her laugh more than anybody else, too. So whether it's bringing home a favorite comedy

video, Elvis "Love Me Tender" shampoo, or underwear with gold studs and darts, do it for laughs. This says: "I want to cheer you up and I'm willing to do anything it takes."

- Set aside special together time once a day. Cancer is an emotional experience that changes from day to day. Make a point of having one special time each day to check in with each other. How is s/he feeling today? How are *you* doing? How are kids faring? Many couples find that staying in bed an extra 10 to 15 minutes each morning to hold each other and talk is a good time to do this.
- Let the ill partner set the pace. The ill partner can guide the pace of the day by how s/he's feeling. This doesn't mean that a spouse or partner shouldn't share his/her feelings but that s/he should take extra care to respond to what the ill partner is feeling.
- Support your partner if s/he wants to talk about the cancer with your friends. People have different ways of coping, and some really choose to be more open about their illness. So if s/he wishes to talk about her cancer, don't feel as though you have to hide the fact that there is cancer in your house. As discussed in chapter 3, this may make some friends uncomfortable, but many others will become better and closer friends as a result.

What a Life Partner Is Going through

Counselors who work with cancer patients often note that it's unfortunate more research into the partner's feelings isn't done. There are some universal feelings of anxiety and angst a spouse will go through. If you're in this position, awareness and acknowledgment that you're not alone in these feelings is the first step in coping with them:

- Sleeplessness. Waking up at 2:00 in the morning in a panic, where all you're thinking about is the cancer is a common experience. Sharing this problem with your ill partner as well as a counselor is a healthy way of dealing with it.
- Separation anxiety. You may suddenly have a tremendous need to spend more time with the ill partner and miss her or him terribly when s/he's not with you. This is a normal reaction when you're facing a life-threatening illness.
- Not wanting to talk about your feelings. This is most common with male partners, who typically learn in our culture to cope with feelings by burying them. "Take it like a man" is one adage that doesn't work

here. As one husband said: "If you don't talk, it *still* won't go away!" Going to spousal support groups where you can meet other men in the same circumstance is the best way to cope with this.

- Feeling that the ill partner is "wallowing" in his/her cancer. A person going through cancer may want to talk about it openly—over and over again. S/he may want to rehash discussions you had yesterday, last week or last month. You may feel as though it's not necessary to keep discussing the cancer or treatment, but this need to constantly discuss it is how many integrate the experience. Be patient. When a person does this, it's also a sign that s/he feels close enough with you to share.
- Feeling left out. Friends and acquaintances will begin to call in after surgery and during treatment to see how the ill partner is doing, sometimes completely ignoring the well partner's feelings. This can cause the well partner to feel ignored, resentful and not appreciated for all the caregiving s/he's doing. Sharing these feelings with the ill partner or a counselor is the best way to work through it.
- Feeling differently about sex. This is especially true after RAI therapy, where there may be fears associated with intimacy.

Avoiding Intimacy

Couples who've gone through RAI therapy acknowledge that avoiding intimacy is one of the "tricks" couples use to avoid the fear of re-establishing contact—particularly if the dosage was high. One of two scenarios takes place. In the first one, the ill partner is feeling better and busies him or herself with so many things s/he just "never has time" for sex anymore. S/he's in bed late, is exhausted and is up early to start all over again the next day.

In the second scenario, the well partner is so relieved that the ill partner is taking over his or her role in the household again, he or she appears to forget about the cancer, trying to put it behind them, and never wanting to discuss the experience again, which greatly interferes with the couple's intimacy.

Couples who've been through these scenarios recommend:

- Spending more "slowed down" time together. Go to bed earlier at night or stay in bed later in the morning to talk and cuddle. Go for more walks, and so on.
- If the ill partner (who's now well) is spending too much time away from the well partner, let him or her know. Tell them you miss them.
- Making dates with each other. Lunch dates, dinner dates, and so on. Courtship is an important part of re-establishing intimacy.

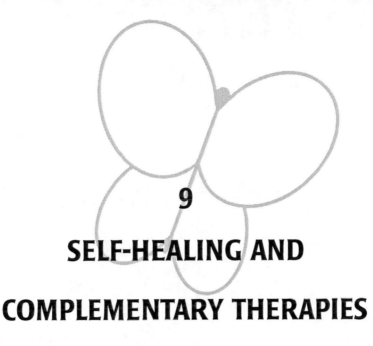

9

SELF-HEALING AND

COMPLEMENTARY THERAPIES

While you're undergoing treatment for thyroid cancer, there are a myriad of self-healing strategies and complementary therapies you can incorporate into your treatment, which may improve your well-being and overall health. This chapter is a general overview, culled from some of my other books in this area. You may find that your own physicians are not supportive of complementary therapies. Doctors make the mistake of assuming that "complementary" is synonymous with "alternative" and worry that their patients may abandon clearly curative therapies in the hopes that drinking a Chinese tea will cure their thyroid cancer. On the other hand, keep in mind that "natural" is not necessarily "not harmful" and many conscientious physicians require a higher standard of scientific evidence before recommending complementary therapies that have not been evaluted in this fashion. What I mean by "complementary," is that you can "have RAI and a massage, too!" As one thyroid cancer survivor stated to me: "It's not possible to write a book on cancer in this century without including information on complementary therapies; people are starved for it." More than 90 percent of cancer patients surf the Internet for this information, which is why I felt a moral obligation to provide this content. I encourage all my readers to search quackwatch.com as well as the alternative medicine archive maintained by the American Cancer Society. See the Resources at the back of this books to links.

Boosting Your Immune System

It's common for people undergoing cancer treatment or awaiting cancer treatment to have a lowered immunity. Part of this is due to stress, which lowers the immune system. In addition, our bodies may be trying to fight the cancer cells. Prior to my own thyroid cancer diagnosis, I fought a cold for an entire year; it simply wouldn't go away. But there are a number of things you can do to boost your immunity and avoid colds and flu.

Avoiding Colds

If you know someone who has a cold, avoid touching him or her, and wash your hands before you touch your nose or eyes. There are also a number of herbal treatments that can stop a cold before it starts, or fully "implodes" in your body.

- Zinc. Available as a lozenge, one of these dissolved under the tongue at the first sign of a cold can stop it in its tracks, according to years of anecdotal reports. (I, too, have great success using zinc.) A study published in the *Annals of Internal Medicine* that looked at zinc lozenges and the common cold in 48 patients showed that zinc lozenges cut the severity and duration of the cold down by almost 50 percent. Not all studies on zinc show the same results, but there are problems with the way many studies looking at herbal products are designed.
- Echinacea. Available in gel caps, tea, and extract, this is a popular prophylactic (meaning "preventative") cold remedy. Anecdotal evidence shows that taking echinacea at the first sign of a cold can either stop it before it becomes full-blown, or shorten its duration. Studies looking at echinacea are difficult to design because there are three difference species of echinacea used as herbal medicines. Echinacea is also available in different preparations and strengths.
- Zinc nasal spray (sold by the brand name, Zicam). A study of 213 patients published in *ENT*, the *Ear, Nose and Throat Journal*, found that cold symptoms were reduced by as much as 75 percent.

Avoiding Flu

When you're immune-suppressed, you're vulnerable to influenza, or the "flu." In a new era of bioterrorism, you may be inclined to shrug off the flu as not that serious compared to other infectious agents, but each year about 20,000 North Americans die because of flu-related pneumonia; about 90 percent of those deaths occur in the frail or elderly.

If you've been hit with a flu in the past, you know how miserable it can be. Generally, the flu vaccine (a.k.a. flu shot) is recommended to certain populations of people (see below). People who are immune-suppressed are always advised to get a flu shot. If you've never had a flu shot, and never seem to get the flu, you may not need to be vaccinated. But if you're undergoing a period of high stress, you may benefit from getting a flu vaccine.

The flu is essentially a respiratory tract infection that hits urban populations in the late fall, winter or early spring. It's very contagious, and spreads person-to-person through mists or sprays—emitted from coughing and sneezing. In 1918, one bad strain of the flu caused over 20 million deaths worldwide and 500,000 deaths in the United States. And the 1968 "Asian Flu" was responsible for over 50,000 deaths in the United States.

When you have the flu, you feel really sick. You may develop a sudden fever as high as 104° F, with shaking chills, muscle and joint aches, sweating, dry cough, nasal congestion, sore throat, and headache. Severe fatigue and just feeling horrible in general (called "malaise") always accompanies these symptoms. The flu can keep you down for as long as two weeks; if you're lucky, you'll escape with a single week. The main complication of the flu is pneumonia, which is what people end up dying from when they're very frail or elderly.

If you want to avoid the flu, ask your doctor about getting a flu vaccine. People who should not be vaccinated are those with an allergy to chicken eggs; a previous bad reaction to the flu vaccine; or those who are currently ill with a fever. Generally, the following groups of people are always advised to get a flu vaccine by both the U.S. and Canadian flu advisory experts:

- Anyone over 65 (the U.S. recommends anyone over 50).
- Anyone living in a nursing home or long-term care facility.
- Anyone with chronic heart and lung diseases, including asthma and kidney disease.
- Anyone with diabetes.
- Anyone who is immune-suppressed or immune-compromised, due to cancer treatment, HIV, organ transplants, steroid medications.
- All health care workers.

The Thyroid Cancer Book

- Anyone caring for someone vulnerable to the flu.
- Children aged 6 months to 18 years who are receiving long-term aspirin therapy (the flu in this case can lead to Reye syndrome, a rare disorder).
- Pregnant women in the second or third trimester during flu season.
- Anyone traveling abroad.

There are now also a number of homeopathic flu-prevention therapies you can ask your natural pharmacist about.

Allergies and Asthma

Lowered immunity can also worsen or trigger allergies and asthma. There are a number of homeopathic and naturopathic allergy treatments available, but they vary greatly, and are dependent on so many factors. These factors, when combined with the range in your actual allergy symptoms, make it impossible to adequately discuss them here. A naturopathic or homeopathic practitioner will assess your lifestyle, diet, and overall exposure to various allergens before suggesting a remedy.

There are essential oils that also help with allergies, the most popular of which is peppermint oil. If you're sneezing, and congested, peppermint oil can be diffused in a room, or applied directly to (this sounds weird) the nape of your neck, as well as the front of your thymus gland (at the indent in your neck at the front) and the soles of your feet. Do not apply peppermint oil to your nose or face as it's very strong and can greatly irritate the skin. You can also apply a few drops of peppermint oil to a hot bath. If you're allergic to dust mites, you can use peppermint oil as a dusting oil, and apply it to wood—especially effective around your bed.

OTC Allergy Medications

Again, many people survive allergies by taking over-the-counter antihistamines. BUT MANY OF THESE CONTAIN IODINE. So check first with your doctor before you purchase these. An antihistamine inhibits what's called a histamine, which is a natural inflammatory substance our bodies make. Histamine is what causes us to sneeze, drip, and even cough. It's not always a bad thing, and it's important not to use antihistamines for prolonged periods of time.

If you tend to suffer from allergies in sealed environments with poor air circulation, taking an antihistamine prior to airplane travel can save you from the pain of clogged sinus passages during take-off and landings.

The first generation of antihistamines is sedating—better for colds than allergies. The second generation of antihistamines—non-sedating—is what most people are taking today for allergies.

The sedating antihistamines are dangerous if you're trying to maintain other activities.

Natural Immune Boosters

Since stress and cancer lower our resistance to disease by suppressing our immune systems, here's an overview of some of the anecdotal information about immune boosters that will help to stimulate your immune system or strengthen it to help fight diseases, including cancer:

1. *Echinacea.* Also mentioned under herbal cold cures, echinacea is not just for colds. This is a flower that belongs to the sunflower family. It's believed that echinacea increases the number of cells in your immune system to fight off diseases of all sorts.

2. *Essiac.* This is a mixture of four herbs comprising Indian rhubarb, sheepshead sorrel, slippery elm, and burdock root. Essiac is believed to strengthen the immune system; improve appetite; supply essential nutrients to the body; possibly relieve pain; and ultimately, prolong life.

3. *Ginseng.* This is a root used in Chinese medicine, but it's believed to enhance your immune system and boost the activity of white blood cells.

4. *Green Tea.* This is a popular Asian tea made from a plant called camellia sinensis. The active chemical in green tea is epigallocatechin gallate (EGCG). It's believed that green tea neutralizes free radicals, which are carcinogenic. It's considered to be an anti-cancer tea—particularly for stomach, lung, and skin cancers.

5. *Iscador* (a.k.a. mistletoe). Iscador is made through a fermentation process, using different kinds of mistletoe, a plant known for its white berries. More popular as an anti-tumor treatment in Europe, it's believed that iscador works by enhancing your immune system and inhibiting tumor growth.

6. *Paul d'Arco* (a.k.a. taheebo). This usually comes in the form of a tea made from the inner bark of a tree called tabebuia. It's believed to a cleansing agent and can be used as an antimicrobial agent, and is said to stop tumor growth.

7. *Wheatgrass.* This is grass grown from wheatberry seeds, which are rich in chlorophyll. Its juice contains over 100 vitamins, minerals,

and nutrients and is believed to contain a number of cancer-fighting agents and immune-boosting properties.

The following spices are said to be "tumor busters" in the alternative health press:

- garlic
- turmeric
- onions
- black pepper
- asfetida
- pippali
- cumin and poppy seeds
- kandathiipile
- neem flowers
- mananthakkali, drumstick, and basil leaves
- ponnakanni
- parsley

Amazing Grapes

A March 2002 study, published by researchers at the Clinical Research Institute at Albany Medical College, tested cell lines for papillary thyroid carcinoma and follicular thyroid carcinoma, and determined that treatment with *resveratrol* activated the cells' "self-destruct" properties, helping to kill them. Resveratrol is an antioxidant found primarily in the skin of red grapes that is known to affect the stickiness of blood platelets and reduce inflammation. This research was performed in cell cultures and may have dietary implications if verified in future clinical trials, but still has not been tested in animals or humans. At any rate, a glass of red wine is harmless at best when you're not hypothyroid.

Discover Your Life Force Energy

All ancient, non-Western cultures, be they in native North America, India, China, Japan or ancient Greece, believed that there were two fundamental aspects to the human body. There was the actual physical shell (clinically called the corporeal body), that makes cells, blood, tissue and so on, and then there was an energy flow that made the physical body come alive. This was known as the life force or life energy. In fact, it was so central to the view of human function that every non-Western culture has a word for "life force." In China, it's called *qi* (pronounced chee); in India it's called *prana*; in Japan it's called *ki*, while the ancient Greeks called it *pneuma* (which has become a prefix in medicine having to do with breath and lungs).

Today, Western medicine concentrates on the corporeal body and doesn't recognize that we have a life force. However, in non-Western, ancient healing, it's thought that the life force is what heals the corporeal body—not the other way around!

Incorporating the concept of life force, non-Western healers look upon the parts of the body as "windows" or "maps" to the body's health. In Chinese medicine, the ears are a complex map, with each point on the ear representing a different organ and part of the psyche. In reflexology, it's the feet that are "read" in order to learn more about the rest of the body and spirit. In the Ayurveda, the tongue is read, while other traditions read the iris of the eyes, and so on. Western medicine doesn't really do this. Instead it looks at every individual part for symptoms of a disease and treats that part individually. So, let's say you notice blurred vision. You might go to an eye doctor and be given a prescription for glasses and be sent on your way. But if this same person were to go to a Chinese medicine doctor, she'd be told that the degeneration of her eyes point to an unhealthy liver. To a Chinese medicine doctor, the eyes are a direct window into the liver. (Interestingly, it's the eyes that turn yellow when you're jaundiced.) So instead of a simple prescription for glasses, the Chinese healer would look into deeper causes of this liver imbalance in the body. You'd be asked about your personal relationships, your diet, your emotional well-being, and your job. And, the treatment may involve a host of dietary changes, stress-relieving exercises and herbal remedies. An Ayurvedic doctor may use the tongue to diagnose a liver imbalance, but the approach is the same. You'd be asked about your diet, lifestyle, work habits, and so on. In other words, the body isn't seen as separate from the self. And to a non-Western healer, what makes us who we are basically has to do with our individual personalities and our societal roles: who we marry, where we work and so on, and how we *feel* about those things are just as important as our visual problems.

One of the most ancient forms of healing involves energy healing, which can involve therapeutic touch or healing touch. Technically, these techniques are considered forms of biofield therapy. An energy healer will use his or her hands to help guide your life force energy. The hands may rest on the body, or just close to the body, not actually touching it. Energy healing is used to reduce pain and inflammation, improve sleep patterns, appetite, and reduce stress. Energy healing, supported by the American Holistic Nurses Association, has been incorporated into conventional nursing techniques with good results. Typically, the healer will move loosely cupped hands in a symmetric fashion on your body, sensing cold, heat, or vibration. The healer will then place his or her hands over areas where the life force energy is imbalanced in order to restore and regulate the energy flow.

All forms of hands-on healing work in some way with the life force energy. Therapies that help to move or stimulate the life force energy include:

- Healing touch
- Tuana
- Mari-el
- Qi gong
- Reiki
- SHEN therapy
- Therapeutic touch

Massage

For many, dramatic emotional wellness is at their fingertips! Massage therapy can be beneficial whether you're receiving the massage from your spouse or a massage therapist trained in any one of dozens of techniques from shiatsu to Swedish massage. In the East, massage was extensively written about in *The Yellow Emperor's Classic of Internal Medicine*, published in 2,700 BC (the text that frames the entire Chinese medicine tradition). In Chinese medicine, massage is recommended as a treatment for a variety of illnesses; tuana massage, a form of deep tissue massage, combined with acupuncture is very effective. A Swedish doctor and poet, Per Henrik, who borrowed techniques from ancient Egypt, China and Rome, developed Swedish massage, the method Westerners are used to experiencing, in the 19th Century.

It's out of shiatsu in the East and Swedish massage in the West that all the many forms of massage were developed. While the philosophies and styles differ in each tradition, the common element is the same: to mobilize the natural healing properties of the body, which will help it maintain or restore optimal health. Shiatsu-inspired massage focuses on balancing the life force energy; Swedish-inspired massage works on more physiological principles. It relaxes muscles to improve blood flow throughout connective tissues, which ultimately strengthens the cardiovascular system.

Massage is more technically referred to as soft tissue manipulation. But no matter what kind of massage you have, there exist numerous, helpful gliding and kneading techniques used along with deep circular movements and vibrations that will relax muscles, improve circulation and increase mobility. All are known to help relieve stress and, often, ease muscle and joint pain. In fact, a number of employers cover massage therapy in their health plans. Massage is becoming so popular that the number of licensed massage therapists enrolled in the American Massage Therapy Association has grown from 1,200 in 1983 to more than 38,000 today. (To find a licensed massage therapist, see the resources at the back of this book.)

Some benefits of massage include:

- Improved circulation
- Improved lymphatic system
- Faster recovery from musculoskeletal injuries
- Soothed aches and pains
- Reduced edema (water retention)
- Reduced anxiety

Types of massage include:

- Deep tissue massage
- Manual lymph drainage
- Neuromuscular massage
- Sports massage
- Swedish massage
- Shaitsu massage

Yoga

Yoga is not just about various stretches or postures, but is actually a way of life for many. It is part of a whole science of living known as the Ayurveda. The Ayurveda is an ancient Indian approach to health and wellness that's stood up quite well to the test of time (it's roughly 3,000 years old). Essentially, it divides up the universe into three basic constitutions or "energies" known as *doshas*. The three *doshas* are based on wind (*vata*), fire (*pitta*) and earth (*kapha*). These *doshas* also govern our bodies, personalities and activities. When our *doshas* are balanced, all functions well, but when they're not balanced, a state of disease (dis-ease as in "not at ease") can set in. Finding the balance involves changing your diet to suit your predominant *dosha* (foods are classified as *kapha*, *vata* or *pitta* and we eat more or less of whatever we need for balance) and practicing yoga, which is a preventative health science that involves certain physical postures, exercises, and meditation. Essentially, yoga is the "exercise" component of Ayurveda. And is designed to tone and soothe your mental state and physical state. Most people benefit from introductory yoga classes, or even introductory yoga videos.

Pressure Point Therapies

Pressure point therapies involve using the fingertips to apply pressure to pressure points on the body. They're believed to help reduce stress, anxiety, pain, and other physical symptoms of stress or other ailments. There are different kinds of pressure point therapies; one of the best known is acupuncture and reflexology.

Acupuncture is an ancient Chinese healing art, which aims to restore the smooth flow of life energy (*qi*) to the body. Acupuncturists believe that your *qi* can be accessed from various points on your body, such as your ear. And each point is associated with a specific organ. So depending on your physical health, an acupuncturist will use a fine needle on a very specific point to restore *qi* to various organs. Each of the roughly 2,000 points on your body has a specific therapeutic effect when stimulated. Acupuncture can relieve many of the physical symptoms and ailments caused by stress; it's now believed that acupuncture stimulates the release of endorphins, which is why it's effective in reducing stress, anxiety, pain and so forth.

Western reflexology was developed by Dr. William Fitzgerald, an American ear, nose and throat specialist, who described reflexology as "zone therapy." But in fact reflexology is practiced in several cultures, including Egypt, India, Africa, China and Japan. In the same way as the ears are a map to the organs in Chinese medicine, with valuable pressure points that stimulate the life force, here the feet play the same role. By applying pressure to certain parts of the feet, hands, and even ears, reflexologists can ease pain and tension and restore the body's life force energy. Like most Eastern healing arts, reflexology aims to release the flow of energy through the body along its various pathways. When this energy is trapped for some reason, illness can result. When the energy is released, the body can begin to heal itself. A reflexologist views the foot as a microcosm of the entire body. Individual reference points or reflex areas on the foot correspond to all major organs, glands, and parts of body. Applying pressure to a specific area of the foot stimulates the movement of energy to the corresponding body part.

Shiatsu massage also involves using pressure points. A healer using Shiatsu will travel the length of each energy pathway (also called meridian), applying thumb pressure to successive points along the way. The aim is to stimulate acupressure points while giving you some of his/her own life energy. Barefoot shiatsu involves the healer using his foot instead of hand to apply pressure. Jin shin jyutsu and jin shin do are other pressure point therapies similar to acupuncture.

You can learn to work your own pressure points, too. Here are some simple pressure point exercises you can try:

1. With the thumb of one hand, slowly work your way across the palm of the other hand, from the base of the baby finger to the base of the index finger. Then rub the center of your palm with your thumb. Push on this point. This will calm your nervous system. Repeat this using the other hand.

2. To relieve a headache, grasp the flesh at the base of one thumb with the opposite index finger and thumb. Squeeze gently and massage the tissue in a circular motion. Then, pinch each fingertip. Switch to the other hand.

3. For general stress relief, find sore pressure points on your feet and ankles. Gently press your thumb into them, and work each sore point. The tender areas are signs of stress in particular parts of your body. By working them, you're relieving the stress and tension in various organs, glands and tissues. You can also apply pressure with bunched and extended fingers, the knuckles, the heel of the hand, or by using the entire hand in a gripping motion.

4. For self-massage of the hands, use the above techniques, paying special attention to tender points on the palms and wrists.

5. Use the above technique to self-massage the ears. Feel for tender spots on the flesh of the ears and work them with vigorous massage. Within about four minutes the ears will get very hot.

Aromatherapy

Essential oils, comprised from plants (mostly herbs and flowers), can do wonders to relieve stress naturally; many essential oils are known for their calming and antidepressant effects. The easiest way to use essential oils is in a warm bath; you simply drop a few drops of the oil into the bath, and sit and relax in it for about 10 minutes. The oils can also be inhaled (put a few drops in a bowl of hot water, lean over with a towel over your head and breathe); diffused (using a lamp ring, or a ceramic diffuser—that thing that looks like a fondue pot.); or sprayed into the air as a mist. The following essential oils are known to have calming, sedative, and/or antidepressant effects: ylang ylang, neroli, jasmine, orange blossom, cedarwood, lavender (a few drops on your pillow will also help you sleep), chamomile, marjoram, geranium, patchouli, rose, sage, clary sage, and sandalwood.

The following scents are considered stimulating and energizing: lemon, grapefruit; peppermint, rosemary, and pine. See my aromatherapy chart to combat hypothyroid symptoms in *The Hypothyroid Sourcebook*.

Qi Gong

Every morning, all over China, people of all ages gather at parks to do their daily Qi gong exercises. Pronounced "Ch'i Kung," these are exercises that help get your life force energy flowing and unblocked. Qi gong exercises are modeled after movements in wildlife (such as birds or animals), movement of trees and other things in nature. The exercises have a continuous flow, rather than the stillness of a posture seen in yoga. Using the hands in various positions to gather in the *qi,* move the *qi,* or release the *qi* is one of the most important aspects of Qi gong movements.

One of the first group of Qi gong exercises you might learn are the "seasons"—fall, winter, spring, summer and late summer (there are five seasons here). These exercises look more like a dance with precise, slow movements. The word *qi* means vitality, energy and life force; the word "*gong*" means practice, cultivate, refine. The Chinese believe that practicing Qi gong balances the body, and improves physical and mental well-being. These exercises push the life force energy into the various meridian pathways that correspond to organs, incorporating the same map used in pressure point healing. Qi gong improves oxygen flow, and enhances the lymphatic system. Qi gong is similar to Tai Chi, except it allows for greater flexibility in routine. The best place to learn Qi gong is through a qualified instructor. You can generally find Qi gong classes through the alternative healing community. Check health food stores and other centers that offer classes such as yoga or Tai Chi. Qi gong is difficult to learn from a book or video, so an instructor is best.

Feng Shui

Pronounced "fung shway" this is the ancient practice of creating energy and harmony through your environmental surroundings (landscaping, interior design, and architecture). People tend to think of feng shui as something that can bring wealth to you (as in money corners) or romance (as in hanging certain items over the bed), but this is in fact not what authentic feng shui consultants look for. Harmony has many elements to it, and where you live, how you live, and a host of other geographic surroundings can all affect how to arrange your environment. Feng shui consultants will assess the following:

1. Entrance. How is it lit? What do you have at your entrance (flowers, chimes, or a stack of old newspapers)?
2. Grounds. What kinds or colors of flowers are around your home? Are there rocks or sculpture around the grounds of your home?
3. Specific areas inside your home. These include your work space/home office, "chef station" or kitchen, bedroom, bathroom, and so on. Placement of mirrors, pictures, plants, lamps, candles, rugs, furniture, bed or even aquariums, are all considered significant. For example, round mirrors or octagonal mirrors are powerful.

In general, feng shui tries to optimize your outdoor spaces through the use of curvilinear and rectangular visual contours or edges; wildlife; landscaping/vegetation; aquatic habitat, and minimizing things that interfere with harmony such as signage, power lines, etc. Inside the home, live plants, colors, lighting, and the positioning of furniture to maximize views of natural scenery are important. Feng shui is said to reduce stress, blood pressure, and lower adrenaline levels. Beginning with a book on feng shui is a good primer—there are dozens of these!

Meditation

Meditation simply requires you to *stop thinking* (about your life, problems, etc.) and *just be*. To do this, people usually find a relaxing spot, or sit quietly and breathe deeply for a few minutes. There is also what I call "active meditation" that can include:

- Taking a walk or hike
- Swimming
- Running or jogging
- Gardening
- Playing golf
- Listening to music
- Dancing
- Reading for pleasure
- Walking your dog
- Practicing breathing exercises (or simply listening to the sounds of your own breathing)
- Practicing stretching exercises
- Practicing yoga or Qi gong

Calm Your Nerves

There are a variety of "nerve herbs" available over the counter at most drug stores or natural health stores. An herb that is said to be "nervine" means that it has a positive effect on the nervous system. It could be toning, relaxing, stimulating, antidepressant, or analgesic. Many people find the following herbal supplements helpful in combating the range of emotional symptoms that the stress of cancer can create, such as irritability, anxiety, sleeplessness and mild to moderate depression:

- *St. John's Wort.* Also known as hypericum, this has been used as a sort of "nerve tonic" in folk medicine for centuries. It's been shown to successfully treat mild to moderate depression and anxiety. It's been used in Germany for years as a first-line treatment for depression, and was endorsed by the American Psychiatric Association in the mid-1990s. In Germany and other parts of Europe, it outsells Prozac prescriptions. Since it was introduced into North America in the early 1990s, millions of North Americans began using St. John's Wort; in the United States, sales of St. John's Wort and other botanical products reached an estimated $4.3 billion dollars in 1998, according to *Nutrition Business Journal*. The benefit of St. John's Wort is that it has minimal side effects, can be mixed with alcohol, is non-addictive, and doesn't require a periodic increase in dosage as with antidepressants. You can go on and off of St. John's Wort as you wish, without any problem; it helps you sleep and dream; it doesn't have any sedative effect, and in fact enhances your alertness. Recently, many studies have come out against St. John's Wort, mainly suggesting it has no real benefitsand may interfere with other prescription drugs, particularly drugs administered to people with AIDS or certain types of cancers. Thus, if you're considering taking St. John's Wort, discuss the potential side effects with your herbalist, pharmacist, or doctor. Then weigh the side effects reported with St. John's Wort against the long list of major side effects reported with antidepressants.That's the only way to make an informed choice. There's nothing harmful with a *start low, go slow* approach.

- *Kava Root.* From the black pepper family, another popular herb is kava (Piper methysticum), which has been a popular herbal drink in the South Pacific for centuries. Kava grows on the islands of Polynesia, and is known to calm nerves, ease stress, fatigue, and anxiety, which results in an antidepressant effect. Kava can also help alleviate migraine headaches and menstrual cramps. Placebo-controlled studies conducted by the National Institute of Mental Health showed that kava significantly relieved anxiety and stress, without the problem of dependency or addiction to the herb. Kava shouldn't be combined with alcohol because it can make the effects of alcohol more potent. Some studies have now shown that excessive use of kava root can lead to liver damage. You should also check with your doctor before you combine kava with any prescription medications.
- *SAM-e.* Pronounced "Sammy," this is another natural compound shown to help alleviate anxiety and mild depression. Since it was introduced in the United States in March 1999, more people have purchased Sam-e than St. John's Wort. Sam-e has also been shown to help relieve joint pain and improve liver function, which makes it popular for the people suffering from arthritis as well. Sam-e stands for S-adenosylmethionine, a compound made by your body's cells. Studies done in Italy during the 1970s documented Sam-e's effectiveness as an antidepressent; recent U.S. studies confirm those results. Some people have reported hot, itchy ears as a side effect.

- *Ginkgo*. This is a plant used to treat a variety of ailments, and is a common herb in Chinese medicine. It can improve memory, and some studies show that it can boost the effectiveness of antidepressant medications.
- *Valerian Root*. This is similar to kava root in that it works as an antianxiety agent, as well as combatting insomnia. When you combine valerian root with passion flower oatstraw or chamomile, the result is relaxing, toning, and restorative.
- *Ginseng*. This helps you adapt better to stress (physical or psychological). It's also thought to boost the immune system.
- *Astragalus*. Similar to ginseng, this Chinese herb helps your body adapt to stress by strengthening the immune system.

Counseling

If you're experiencing depression, anxiety or panic, or are experiencing problems with your family or partner (see previous chapter) one of the best things you can do is to talk to a professional. Simply finding someone to talk to—someone who is objective—can make an enormous difference. Most people looking for "sorting out your life" counseling do well with counselors or social workers, but the following professionals can all help:

- Psychologist or Psychological Associate: This is someone who can be licensed to practice therapy with either a master's degree or doctoral degree. Clinical psychologists have a Masters of Science degree (MSc.) or Master of Arts (MA), and will usually work in a hospital or clinic setting, but often can be found in private practice. Clinical psychologists can also hold a Ph.D. (Doctor of Philosophy) in psychology, an Ed.D. (Doctor of Education) or, if they're American, a Psy.D. (Doctor of Psychology).
- Social Worker: This professional holds a BSW (Bachelor of Social Work), and/or a MSW (Master of Social Work), having completed a Bachelor's degree in another discipline (which is not at all uncommon). Some social workers have Ph.D.s as well. A professional social worker has a degree in social work and meets state legal requirements. The designation "CSW" stands for Certified Social Worker. It's a legal title granted by the state. A designation of ACSW refers to the National Association of Social Workers' (NASW) own, non-

governmental national credential and stands for the "Academy of Certified Social Workers." Unlike the CSW, which, in addition to the exam, requires graduation (in most states) from a masters level program, the ACSW requires two years of supervised experience following graduation from such a program. Some social workers have a "P" and "R": these letters stand for CSWs who have become qualified under state law to receive insurance reimbursement for outpatient services to clients with group health insurance. Each initial refers to a different type of insurance policy. The "P" requires three years of supervised experience, while the "R" requires six years.

- Psychiatric Nurse: This is most likely a registered nurse (R.N.) with a bachelor of science in nursing (BSc.) (which isn't absolutely required) who probably has, but doesn't necessarily require, a master's degree in nursing, too. The master's degree could be either an MA (Master of Arts) or an MSc. (Master of Science). This nurse has done most of his or her training in a psychiatric setting, and *may* be trained to do psychotherapy.

- Counselor: This professional has *usually* completed certification courses in counseling, and therefore has obtained a license to practice psychotherapy; s/he may have, but doesn't require, a university degree. Frequently, though, counselors will have a master's degree in a related field, such as social work. Or, they may have a master's degree in a field having nothing to do with mental health. The term "professional counselor" is used to represent those persons who have earned a minimum of a master's degree and possess professional knowledge and demonstrable skills in the application of mental health, psychological, and human development principles in order to facilitate human development and adjustment throughout the life span. As of January 1999, the District of Columbia and 44 states have enacted some type of counselor credentialing law, which regulates the use of titles related to the counseling profession. The letters "CPC" stand for Certified Professional Counselor, and refer to the title granted by the state legislative process. The letters "LPC" stand for Licensed Professional Counselor, and refer to the most often granted state statutory counselor credential. No matter what letters you see, however, it's always a good idea to ask your counselor what training s/he's had in the field of mental health.

- Marriage and Family Counselor: This is somewhat different than the broader term "counselor." This professional has completed rigorous training through certification courses in family therapy and relationship dynamics, and has obtained a license to practice psychotherapy. This professional should have the designations MFT or AAFMT. MFTs have graduate training (a master's or doctoral degree) in marriage and family therapy and at least two years of clinical experience. There are 41 states currently licensing, certifying or regulating MFTs.

RESOURCES

Note: Some professional thyroid associations are concerned with the accuracy of information about thyroid cancer and thyroid disease you may find on the Internet. To help wade through the "wild" information you may find out there, I encourage all of my readers to contact the American Thyroid Association (*www.thyroid.org*) to verify Internet information or health claims.

You can also visit the vast alternative medicine archive run by the American Cancer Society:

http://www.cancer.org/docroot/ETO/ETO_5.asp?sitearea=ETO

Or, take a look at Quackwatch at *www.quackwatch.com*, the website run by Stephen Barrett, M.D., a retired psychiatrist who is vice-president of the National Council Against Health Fraud, and scientific advisor to the American Council on Science and Health. Dr. Barrett welcomes questions and emails to:sbinfo@quackwatch.com.

I encourage readers, too, to get involved with thyroid cancer listservs, and use them to reach out to others, as well as recommend thyroid cancer reading material or links that are particularly helpful!

Thyroid Cancer-Specific Sites

ThyCa, Inc. (The Thyroid Cancer Survivors' Association)
P.O. Box 1545
New York, NY 10159-1545
Tel: 877-588-7904 (toll-free)
Fax: 503-905-9725
www.thyca.org
Email: thyca@thyca.org
Here you'll find local chapters, and links to the following support groups:
Advanced Thyroid Cancer Support Group

Anaplastic Support Group
Caregivers Support Group
Long-Term Survivors Support Group
Medullary Support Group
Pediatric Support Group
Thyca Thyroid Cancer Support Group
America Online Thyroid Cancer Support Group
The Thyroid Cancer Online Email Support Group

Canadian Thyroid Cancer Support Group (Thry'vors), Inc.
P.O. Box 23007
550 Eglinton Ave. West
Toronto, ON M5N 3A8
Tel: 416-487-8267 (9 am–5 pm Monday to Friday)
www.thryvors.org
Email: thryvors@sympatico.ca
To join Thry'vors support listserv, go to:
http://groups.yahoo.com/group/thryvors

The Light of Life Foundation
www.lightoflifefoundation.org

The Head and Neck Cancer Foundation
2345 Yonge St., Suite 700
Toronto, ON M4P 2E5
Tel: 416-324-8178
Fax: 416-324-9021
www.headandneckcanada.com

Johns Hopkins Thyroid Tumor Center
www.thyroid-cancer.net

Thyrogen Website
www.thyrogen.com

Other Thyroid Websites of Interest

www.thyroid.org (American Thyroid Association)
www.aace.com (American Association of Clinical Endocrinologists)
www.hypoparathyroidism.org (If you have calcium problems post-surgery)

www.cancernet.nci.nih.gov (National Cancer Institute)
www.endocrineweb.com
www.thyroidmanager.org
www.thyroid.org (The American Thyroid Association)
www.thyroid.com (Santa Monica Thyroid Diagnostic Center, founded by Dr. Richard B. Guttler)
www.mythyroid.com (Thyroid site maintained by Dr. Daniel J. Drucker)

Websites Founded by Thyroid Patients

Mary Shomon's Thyroid Websites
www.thyroid-info.com
thyroid.about.com

Julia Lawrence's Papillary Thyroid Cancer Site
www.papthyca.com

Megan Stendebach's Thyroid Cancer Site
www.thyroidcancersongs.com

Ruth Fawcett's Thyroid Cancer Page
http://www.thyroidcancer.org.uk/

Linda's Thyroid Cancer Page
http://ourworld.compuserve.com/homepages/Sweetwind/thyca/thyca.htm

General Thyroid Organizations

American Foundation of Thyroid Patients
www.thyroidfoundation.org

Thyroid Foundation of America, Inc.
www.allthyroid.org

Thyroid Foundation of Canada
www.thyroid.ca

Outside North America

(Note: mailing address provided only in the absence of an email address or website url.)

AUSTRALIA
Australian Thyroid Foundation
P.O. Box 186
Westmead, NSW 2145
Australia
Tel: 61 2 9890 6962
Fax: 61 2 9755 7073

UNITED KINGDOM
British Thyroid Foundation
www.british-thyroid-association.org
Email: contact@british-thyroid-association.org

EUROPE
European Thyroid Association
www.eurothyroid.com

DENMARK:
Email: Lis_Larsen@net.dialog.dk

FRANCE
Email: mlhoir@aol.com

GERMANY
www.thyrolink.com

ITALY
Associazione Italiana Basedowiani e Tiroidei
C/O Centro Minerva
7 Via Mazzini 43100
Parma, Italy
Tel: 39 521-207771
Fax: 39 521-207771

NORWAY
Norsk Hypothyreoseforening (NHF)
Aili Mjatvedt, Buskerud fylkeslag
Stasjonsgt. 53, N-3300
Hokksund, Norway

THE NETHERLANDS
Schildklierstichting Nederland Postbus 138 1620
AC Hoorn Holland

SWEDEN
Vastsvenska Patientforeningen for Skoldkortelsjoka
Mejerivalen 8 439 36
Onsala, Sweden
Tel: 46 30 06 39 12
Fax: 46 30 06 39 12

LATIN AMERICA
www.lats.org
Email: acbianco@usp.

REPUBLIC OF GEORGIA
Email: diabet@access.sanet.ge

JAPAN
Thyroid Foundation of Japan (TFJ)
www.hata.ne.jp/tfj/
Email: akasu@kt.rim.or.jp

APPENDIX

The following recipes are reprinted content from *The Light of Life Foundation Cookbook: Great Recipes for an Iodine-Free Diet*. Copyright, 1998, The Light of Life Foundation, *www.lightoflifefoundation.org*.

Thyroid cancer patient and survivor, Joan Shey, founded The Light of Life Foundation in 1997. She kindly granted me permission to reprint this wonderful cookbook. I have made only minor editorial changes for clarity and consistency, and have added an asterisk (*) to indicate minor ingredient substitutes, in light of changes to the LID since this cookbook was first written. Many of these recipes are creations of Joan's dear friend Adele, who sadly passed away since this cookbook was produced. The cookbook and this Appendix are dedicated to Adele.

Note: You can use NON-IODIZED salt for any of the following recipes. None of the Light of Life Foundation recipes reprinted here call for salt. For recipes that call for sugar, keep in mind that only white granulated sugar is allowed. No brown sugar is allowed because of its molasses content.

SOUPS

(All soups can be frozen in advance, and reheated when you're hypothyroid.)

Cabbage Soup

> 1 chicken, whole or quartered (optional)
> 1 medium head of white cabbage, quartered, cored and sliced
> 4 medium tomatoes cut into large chunks
> 3 medium carrots, sliced in large pieces
> 2 medium carrots, sliced in large pieces
> 2 medium onions or 2 large leeks, diced (if using leeks, cut in half lengthwise and soak in cold water to cover to make sure there is no sand left in them)
> 2 tablespoons of lemon juice (fresh)
> 2 tablespoons of honey or sugar
> 2 tablespoons of oil (no oil if using chicken)

159

If using chicken, put chicken and onion or leek into water to cover. When it starts to boil, skim dark foam as it forms on the top. After 20 minutes, add remaining ingredients and cook for 30 minutes or until chicken and cabbage are soft enough. Add additional seasoning to make sweeter or tarter. If not using chicken, sauté onion or leek in oil until transparent. Add 6 cups of water. When water comes to a boil, add remaining ingredients. When that boils again, lower heat to simmer for about 40 minutes. Add additional seasoning to taste and check to see if cabbage is soft; it is ready to serve when soft.

Chicken Broth

2 large chickens
2 large onions or 2 leeks, diced
5 carrots sliced in large chunks
small bunch of parsley
pepper to taste

Add chickens and onions to 6 to 8 cups of boiling water. As it boils, skim dark foam off with a slotted spoon. After boiling for about 20 minutes, add remaining ingredients. Boil slowly for about 40 minutes longer uncovered. When chickens are tender, remove from soup. (You can always boil down broth if it's too watery.) Strain (to remove veggies) into 1 or 2 pint containers and keep for other recipes. It can be kept in the freezer for up to 5 months.

Fresh Veggie Soup

All vegetables need to be fresh, not canned.
1 tablespoon canola oil
1 large onion, diced
1 bunch of carrots, diced
1 large parsnip (or white carrot), diced
2 medium potatoes, diced
1 lb mushrooms, sliced
1/2 lb string beans, cut in 1 1/2 inch pieces
1/2 lb green peas
1 lb spinach

1/2 bunch Swiss chard, mustard greens or fresh spinach cut or chopped into large pieces
1/2 head of cabbage, shredded
1 large turnip or rutabaga
2 large tomatoes, peeled and diced
1/2 cup barley and/or brown rice
1 bouquet mixed herbs: parsley, dill, rosemary (tied, with white pepper to taste)

In large stock pot brown onions in oil. Add all of the above and enough water to just about cover the veggies (about 4-6 cups). When it comes to a boil, lower the heat to simmer and cover. Mix ever 15 minutes or so to make sure nothing sticks to the pot. After 45 minutes, when veggies are tender, the soup is ready to serve.

Butternut Squash Soup

2 medium butternut squash, peeled and cut in chunks
2 large sweet potatoes or yams, peeled and cut in chunks
3 large carrots, peeled and cut in chunks
1 medium onion, diced
1 tablespoon of oil
1/2 teaspoon of cinnamon or all spice
white or black pepper to taste
4 cups of water

If you use a food processor you can grate the carrots, squash and sweet potatoes and the soup will be a real purée. It's almost like a cream soup without the cream!

In a large soup pot: sauté the onion in the oil until onions are transparent. Move the pot off the burner and add water. Then move back on burner and when it comes to a boil, add remaining ingredients. Once everything starts to boil, lower the heat to simmer for about an hour, stirring once in a while to make sure nothing sticks to the bottom.

If there are too many chunks of vegetables, and the soup is not smooth enough, put the chunks in the blender and return to the pot.

When serving, sprinkle with a little allspice or cinnamon. If you like the flavors of India, add a touch of cumin or curry to the pot while cooking or when serving.

SALADS

All-purpose salad dressing

    3 large cloves of garlic, minced
    1/3 cup white vinegar
    1/3 cup olive oil
    1/4 cup vegetable oil
    pinch of pepper
    pinch of dried oregano
    pinch of basil

In a medium bowl, add all ingredients except oils. Slowly whisk in oil. Can stay in refrigerator for a week, well covered.

Watercress Salad with Endive and Orange

    1 bunch watercress
    2 Belgian endives
    2 oranges
    1 tablespoon white vinegar
    1 tablespoon extra-virgin olive oil
    freshly ground pepper to taste

Wash the watercress, pat dry and tear into bite-size sprigs. Cut the endives width-wise into 1/4 strips. Cut the rind (both zest and white pith) off the oranges to expose the flesh. Make V-shaped cuts to remove the individual segments from the membranes, working over a large bowl to catch the juice.

Add the vinegar, oil, salt, and pepper to the orange juice in the bowl and whisk until blended. Just before serving, add the watercress, endives, and orange segments. Gently toss to mix and serve at once.

Cucumber Salad with Dill

    2 cucumbers
    3 tablespoons white vinegar
    1 tablespoon sugar
    1 small red onion, sliced and broken into rings
    3 tablespoons finely chopped fresh dill

Wash the cucumbers and partially remove the skin. Peel in lengthwise strips using a vegetable peeler or fork and leaving a little skin between each strip. Thinly slice the cucumber widthwise. Place the vinegar, sugar, pepper (to taste) in a bowl and whisk until the sugar is dissolved. Add the cucumber, onion and dill and toss well. Tastes better when the dressing marinates with the vegetables for about 5 minutes.

Eggplant Salad with Basil

> 3 medium eggplants, about 4 1/2 lbs in all, cut into 1 1/2 cubes (do not peel)
> 1 cup olive oil
> 4 garlic cloves, peeled and minced
> 2 large yellow onions, peeled, halved and thinly sliced
> freshly ground black pepper, to taste
> 1 cup chopped fresh basil leaves, coarsely chopped, juice of 2 lemons

Preheat oven to 400 degrees F. Line a roasting pan with foil and add eggplant. Toss with half of the oil and the minced garlic. Bake for about 35 minutes, until the eggplant is soft but not mushy. Cool slightly and transfer to a large bowl. Heat remaining olive oil in a large skillet. Add sliced onions and cook, covered, over low heat until tender, about 15 minutes. Add onions to the eggplant. Season generously with black pepper; add fresh basil and lemon juice. Toss together. Adjust seasoning and serve at room temperature.

Pineapple Salsa

Can be served with poultry, by itself, or in a pineapple shell.

> 1 small fresh pineapple
> 1 red pepper, cored, seeded, and cut into 1 inch pieces
> 1 yellow pepper, cored, seeded and cut into 1 inch pieces
> 1 green pepper, cored, seeded and cut into 1 inch pieces
> 1 small red onion, finely chopped
> 1/2 cup chopped cilantro
> 3-4 tablespoons fresh lime juice
> Freshly ground pepper
> 1 tablespoon sugar (optional)

Cut the pineapple in half lengthwise. Using a grapefruit knife, cut out the pineapple flesh, leaving the shell intact. Core the pineapple and cut into 1 inch pieces. Combine the pineapple with remaining ingredients in a mixing bowl and gently toss. Correct the seasoning, adding the life juice and sugar to taste. Tastes best when served within 1 hour.

Strawberry-Spinach Salad

   1/4 cup fresh-squeezed orange juice
   1 teaspoon sugar
   1 teaspoon poppy seeds
   1/2 lb fresh spinach
   2 cups fresh, sliced strawberries (orange slices optional)
Combine first three ingredients, stir well and set aside (this is the dressing). Gently tear and toss spinach with strawberries. Arrange in individual plates and drizzle with one tablespoon of the dressing.

PASTA SAUCES

(All can be frozen in advance.)

Basic Tomato Sauce

(Can be served with any pasta; be sure to boil pasta in UNSALTED water, with a little olive oil.) Joan has precooked about a pound of pasta, added this sauce and prepared one-pint containers, which can be taken to the hospital to eat after an RAI treatment. Most hospital staff will happily microwave it and bring it to you.

   2-3 lbs ripe tomatoes, Roma or Beefsteak
   3-4 cloves of garlic, chopped or sliced
   5 leaves of fresh sweet basil or 1/2 teaspoon of dried basil
   1 teaspoon of paprika
   2 tablespoons of olive oil
Blanch tomatoes for 1 minute and then peel and remove seeds and hard core. In a large stockpot, lightly sauté garlic, basil, oregano, and pepper in olive oil for 2-3 minutes. Cut tomatoes into quarters and slowly add to pot of spices. When it comes to

a boil, lower heat to simmer for about 90 minutes, stirring once in a while. Add more spices as needed.

Variations: One large green pepper and one large onion diced can be added to the sauce along with spices and lightly cooked prior to adding tomatoes. If you want to add ground meat (chicken, turkey or beef – WITHOUT PRESERVATIVES), brown the meat along with the spices and then add the tomatoes.

Freezer Tomato Sauce

> 10 large tomatoes, blanched, peeled, seeded and chopped
> 4 cups chopped onions
> 2 cups chopped carrots
> 2 tablespoons chopped fresh Italian (flat leaf) parsley
> 2-3 small garlic cloves, chopped
> 1/2-1 teaspoon oregano leaves, crumbled
> 1-1/2 teaspoons sugar* or granulated sugar substitute
> (Note: Capers, which have iodized salt, have been omitted from the original recipe.)

In 4-quart sauce pan combine all ingredients except sugar or sugar substitute; set over low heat. Bring to simmer and cook until carrots are soft, 30-40 minutes, stirring occasionally to prevent burning. Let cool slightly. In blender container, process 2 cups of tomato mixture until smooth; transfer sauce to 3-quart bowl and repeat procedure with remaining tomato mixture, processing 2 cups at a time. If sauce is slightly bitter, stir in sugar or sugar substitute. Measure sauce into plastic freezer bags or freezer containers and label with date and amount; store in freezer until needed. (Note: Some sugar substitutes cannot be heated; please check with brand/manufacturer label or 800 number.)

Roasted Pepper Sauce

(Best with 3 cups imported penne.)

> 3 large bell peppers (ideally, 1 of each: red, yellow and green)
> 1 small clove garlic, minced (1/2 teaspoon)
> 2 scallions, whites minced, greens finely chopped

1/4 cup finely chopped fresh herbs (basil, oregano, parsley)

3 tablespoons white vinegar

2 teaspoons extra virgin olive oil

2 tablespoons chicken stock (*optional; do NOT use canned chicken stock, only fresh stock– see under Soups)

freshly ground pepper to taste

Boil pasta* in 4 quarts of water until it is al dente (slightly chewy); set aside pasta. Roast the whole peppers over a flame or electric burner until black or charred on all sides. (Alternatively, you can sauté the peppers, garlic and scallions in a pan with a little olive oil.) After roasting or sautéing, take the whole peppers and core and seed them; cut into penne size pieces. Combine the garlic, scallions, and herbs in a large bowl. Add the peppers, vinegar, olive oil, and stock. Stir in the pasta. Correct the seasoning and vinegar to taste.

VEGETABLE SIDE DISHES

A Quick Sauté of Yellow Peppers and Sugar Snap Peas

1 pound fresh sugar snap peas, strung

1 1/2 tablespoons extra virgin olive oil

1 large clove garlic, minced (1 teaspoon)

1/2 teaspoon freshly grated lemon zest

2 yellow or red bell peppers, cored, seeded, and cut into pea pod-size strips

1 tablespoon chopped fresh tarragon, thyme, or basil (1 teaspoon. dried)

Freshly ground peeper to taste

Blanch the peas in 1 quart boiling water for 30 seconds. Drain in a colander and refresh under cold water. Drain and blot dry. Just before serving, heat the oil in a sauté pan. Add the garlic and zest, and cook over medium heat for 30 seconds, or until fragrant. Add the peppers and sauté for 30 seconds. Add the peas, tarragon, and peeper. Cook just long enough to heat the peas. Serve at once.

Mustard Glazed Carrots

2 lbs carrots
3 1/2 tablespoons unsalted margarine*
1/2 teaspoon dry mustard (more to taste)
1/4 cup sugar
Chopped parsley
(For variety, you can add sweet potatoes and oranges)

Scrape and clean carrots and then cut in half lengthwise; cut in half again. Cook carrots until tender. In a small saucepan, melt margarine, add mustard and sugar. Stir until mixture becomes a syrup. Pour over drained carrots. Simmer carrots in mixture for 3 minutes. Sprinkle with parsley and serve.

Roasted Potatoes with Garlic

2 pounds small red potatoes, quartered
2 large garlic cloves, sliced thin
1 1/2 tablespoon olive oil

In a jelly-roll or large baking pan, toss the potatoes with the garlic, the oil, pepper to taste and roast them in the middle of a preheated 500 degrees F oven, stirring once for 30 minutes.

Italian Vegetables

2 tablespoons plus 2 teaspoons reduced margarine (salt free)
2 medium zucchini (about 5 ounces each), cut into 1/4-inch thick slices
1 small eggplant (about 12 ounces), cut into 1/2-inch cubes
1 medium green bell pepper, seeded and cut into thin strips
1/2 cup thinly sliced onion
12 cherry tomatoes, cut into halves
1/2 teaspoon oregano leaves
1/8 teaspoon of garlic powder and pepper, or to taste

In 12 inch non-stick skillet, heat margarine over high heat until bubbly and hot; add zucchini, eggplant, bell peeper and onion and sauté until vegetables are softened, 2 to 3 minutes. Add tomatoes and remaining ingredients and stir to combine thoroughly. Reduce heat to medium-low, cover skillet and cook, stirring occasionally, until vegetables are tender-crisp, 4 to 6 minutes.

Honey-Cinnamon Winter Squash

> 1 butternut squash (about 2 lbs), which will yield about
> 2 cups cooked pulp
> 2 tablespoons each margarine (salt free) and honey
> 1/2 teaspoon each ground cinnamon
> Dash ground nutmeg, or to taste
> 1/2 cup water

Cut squash into half lengthwise and discard seeds and membranes; score cut surface of each squash half in a cross-cross pattern, being careful not to cut through sell. In 10 x10 x2 inch microwave safe baking dish, arrange halves, cut-side up; fill seed cavity of each half with 1 tablespoon margarine evenly with cinnamon and nutmeg and pour water into baking dish; microwave on High until pulp is soft, 10 to 15 minutes longer, basting every 5 minutes. (Cooking times vary depending upon microwave.) To serve, cut each half lengthwise into halves and top each portion with an equal amount of the remaining pan juices.

MEAT DISHES

(Red meat is harder to find without additives or preservatives, so the following recipes are mostly for chicken, which is easier to buy fresh.)

Chicken Francaise

> 4 boneless chicken breasts
> 4 tablespoons olive oil or unsalted margarine
> 1/3 cup chicken broth (see under Soups)
> 1/3 cup lemon juice (fresh)
> Unbleached flour

Lightly bread chicken breast in flour. Heat oil or margarine in frying pan, then add cutlets. Fry until lightly golden, then add chicken broth and lemon. Add sliced mushrooms if you like.

Italian Style Chicken

(Freezes well.)

> 2-3 lbs canned or ripe tomatoes
> 2 1/2 lb chicken, cut into eighths
> 1 cup sliced fresh mushrooms
> 1 cup cut-up onions
> 1 large red or green pepper, cubed
> 2 to 4 cloves minced garlic
> 1 teaspoon oregano
> 2-3 tablespoons of olive oil
> 1 large green or red pepper

Blanch tomatoes for one minute and peel. In a large skillet or oversize frying pan, brown chicken parts in olive oil, pour off 1/2 of the remaining fat. Add oregano, garlic onions and peppers all at the same time. Sauté 5 minutes then add tomatoes (watch for splatters). After cooking about 35 minutes, add the mushrooms. Cover and cook over low heat, simmering about 20-25 minutes. (The cooking time is less if using only breasts: approx. 45 minutes.) May be served over pasta or rice.

Chicken with Orange Pesto

> 1/2 cup fresh basil leaves
> 2 tablespoons grated orange peel
> 2 garlic cloves
> 2 teaspoons olive oil
> 3 tablespoons orange juice
> ground pepper
> 6 chicken breast halves, with skin and bone (about 3 lbs)

Preheat broiler. In food processor, combine basil, orange peel and garlic. Cover and process until finely chopped. Add olive oil, orange juice, and pepper to taste; process a few seconds or until a paste is formed. Lightly spread equal portions of basil mixture under skin and on bone side of each chicken breast. Place chicken, skin-side down, on broiler pan. Broil chicken 4 inches from heat source 10 minutes. Turn chicken over and broil 10 to 12 minutes longer, or until chicken is cooked thoroughly. Cover with foil if chicken begins to brown too quickly.

Chicken and Potatoes with Cinnamon

One 4 lb whole roasting chicken
3 large potatoes or 6 small red potatoes
1 tablespoon canola oil
cinnamon
pepper

Preheat oven to 350 degrees F. Cover roasting pan with oil. Dice a medium onion and place in pan (optional). Place the chicken, breast side down in a pan, and place potatoes, cut in large chunks or whole, if small reds, in roasting pan around chicken. Sprinkle with cinnamon and pepper. Bake with for 45 minutes and then turn potatoes and chicken to breast side up, baste with any juices, and continue cooking for another 45 minutes. When chicken juices run clear, serve.

Fruited Pork Chops

2 pork shoulder or loin chops
1/2 cup thinly sliced carrot
1/3 cup unfermented apple cider (no sugar added)
1/4 cup sliced onion
1/2 small mango, pared, pitted and diced
1/2 small apple, cored and diced
1 cup cooked long-grain rice (hot)
Italian (flat-leaf) parsley sprigs

On rack in broiling pan, broil pork chops 5 inches from heat source, turning once, until rare, 2 to 3 minutes on each side. Remove from broiler and set aside. Preheat oven to 350 degrees F. In 8x8x2 inch baking dish, combine carrot, cider, onion, mango, apple; top with pork chops. Cover and bake until pork chops are fork-tender and vegetables are thoroughly cooked, 30-40 minutes. Serve over hot rice and garnish with parsley.

[Note: Fresh Water Fish recipe has been omitted from original cookbook because currently NO FISH is allowed on the LID.]

SNACKS

Microwave Nutty Apple

> 4 small Red or Golden Delicious Apples, cored
> 2 teaspoons sugar, divided
> 2 tablespoons chunky, unsalted peanut butter (see below)
> Ground cinnamon

Into each of the four 5-ounce custard cups place one apple; sprinkle core cavity of each apple with 1/2 teaspoon sugar, fill each with 1 1/2 teaspoons peanut butter, and top each with 1/4 teaspoon sugar. Sprinkle each apple with an equal amount of cinnamon and microwave on High for 3 to 4 minutes.

Unsalted peanut butter to the rescue:

Joan has added a "post cookbook note" for my readers... For breakfast or snacks, Joan recommends UNSALTED peanut butter, which can be purchased in health or organic food stores. (Please check with the store staff to be sure it is unsalted and natural). Spread it on apples or UNSALTED rice cakes!

* Ingredient changed from original recipe due to LID restrictions.

Bibliography

"Aace/Aaes Medical/Surgical Guidelines for Clinical Practice: Management of Thyroid Carcinoma. Thyroid Carcinoma Task Force." *Endocrine Practice* (Vol 7, No 3) May/June 2001.

Becker, David, M.D. "Radiation and the Thyroid." *Thyrobulletin* (Vol 16, No 3) Autumn 1995.

"Blood Test Detects Thyroid Cancer Gene." *Thyrobulletin* (Vol 16, No 1) Spring 1995.

Bogdanova, Tatyana I., Ph.D., and Nikolaj D. Tranko, M.D., Ph.D. "The Dynamics of Thyroid Cancer in Children in Ukraine after the Chernobyl Accident." Kiev, Ukraine: Institute of Endocrinology and Metabolism, Academy of Medical Sciences of Ukraine. (Unpublished report, compiled 1996.)

Bogner, U. et al. "Association between Thyroid Cytotoxic Antibodies and Atrophic Thyroiditis." *Clinical Thyroidology* (Vol VIII, Issue 1) January-April 1995.

Bunevicius et al. "Effects of Thyroxine as Compared with Thyroxine plus Triiodothyronine in Patients with Hypothyroidism." *The New England Journal of Medicine* (Vol 340, No 6) February 11, 1999, 424-9.

Clark, Orlo H., M.D., and Johann Elmhed. "Thyroid Surgery—Past, Present, and Future." *Thyroid Today* (Vol XVIII, No 1) March 1995.

Cooper, David S., M.D. "Thyroid Nodules and Thyroid Cancer: Evaluation and Treatment." *Thyrobulletin* (Vol 16, No 3) Autumn 1995.

Dickens, B.M. "The Doctrine of Informed Consent" in Ed. Abella, R.S., and M.L. Rothman, *Justice Beyond Orwell.* Montreal: Yvon Blais 1985, 243-63.

Dirusso, G. et al. "Complications of I-131 Radioablation for Well-Differentiated Thyroid Cancer." *Clinical Thyroidology* (Vol VIII, Issue 1) January-April 1995.

Dong B.J. et al. "Bioequivalence of Generic and Brand-Name Levothyroxine Products in the Treatment of Hypothyroidism." *Journal of the American Medical Association* (Vol 277, No 15) April 16, 1997, 277(15):1199-200.

Dottorini, M.E. et al. "Effect of Radioiodine for Thyroid Cancer on Carcinogenesis and Female Fertility." *Clinical Thyroidology* (Vol VIII, Issue 1) January-April 1995.

Emanuel, Ezekiel J. and Linda L. Emanuel. "Four Models of the Physician-Patient Relationship." *Journal of the American Medical Association*(Vol 267, No 16) 1992, 2221-6.

Eskin, B.A. "Effects of Iodine Therapy on Breast Cancer and the Thyroid." Philadelphia, PA: Medical College of Pennsylvania and Hahnemann University. (Abstract from the 6th International Thyroid Symposium, Thyroid and Trace Elements, 1996.)

Etchells, E. et al. "Disclosure." *CMAJ* (Vol 155) 1996, 387-91.

Etchells, E. et al. "Voluntariness." *CMAJ* (Vol 155)1996, 1083-6.

Etchells, E. and Gilbert Sharpe et al. "Consent." *CMAJ* (Vol 155) 1996, 177-80.

Gaz, Randall D., M.D. "Instructions for Patients Undergoing Thyroid Needle Biopsy." *Thyrobulletin* (Vol 14, No 4) Autumn 1993.

Horn-Ross, P.L., A.S. Whittemore, D.W. West, and I. R. McDougall. "Rationale for a Study of Iodine, Selenium and Thyroid Cancer." Union

City, CA: Northern California Cancer Center. (Abstract from the 6th International Thyroid Symposium, Thyroid and Trace Elements, 1996.)

Ito, Masahiro, Shunici Yamashita, Kiyoto Ashizawa, Hiroyuki Namba, Masaharu Hoshi, Yoshisada Shibata, Ichiro Sekine, Shigenobu Nagataki, and Itsuzo Shigematsu. "Childhood Thyroid Diseases around Chernobyl Evaluated by Ultrasound Examination and Fine Needle Aspiration Cytology." *Thyroid* (Vol 5, No 5) 1995.

"Laboratory Tests." Posted to *www.thyca.org*, April 2002.

Levine, R.J. *Ethics and Regulation of Clinical Research.* New Haven: Yale University Press, 1988.

Loebig, Poertl, H.M. Derwahl, H. Schatz, K. Mann, and R. Hoermann. "Regulation of Maternal Thyroid during Pregnancy by Human Chorionic Gonadotropin (hCG)." Bochum, Germany: Essen and Department of Medicine, University of Bochum. (Abstract from the 6th International Thyroid Symposium, Thyroid and Trace Elements, 1996.)

"Low Iodine Diet." Retrieved from *www.thyca.org*, February 2000 and April 2002.

Mastroianni, Anna C., Ruth Faden, and Daniel Federman, Eds. *Women and Health Research: Ethical and Legal Issues of Including Women in Clinical Studies*, Volume 1. Washington: National Academy Press, 1994.

Nygaard, B. et al. "Acute Effects of Radioiodine Therapy on Thyroid Gland Size and Function in Patients with Multi-Nodular Goiter." *Clinical Thyroidology* (Vol VIII, Issue 1) January-April 1995.

Olveira, G. et al. "Altered Bioavailability Due to Changes in the Formulation of a Commercial Preparation of Levothyroxine in Patients with Differentiated Thyroid Carcinoma." *Clinical Endocrinology* (Vol 46) June 1997, 707-11.

O'Riordain, D.S. et al. "Impact of Biochemical Screening of Medullary Thyroid Cancer: Extent of Disease and Outcome in Patients with Multiple Endocrine Neoplasia." *Clinical Thyroidology* (Vol VIII, Issue 1) January-April 1995.

Pellegrino, Edmund D. and D.C. Thomasma. "The Good Physician" in *For The Patient's Good*. New York: Oxford University Press, 1988.

"Radiation." Posted to *www.thyca.org*, April 2002.

Reiners, Chr. "Radioactive Iodine and the Risk of Thyroid Cancer." University of Wurzburg, Germany: Clinic and Policlinic for Nuclear Medicine. (Abstract from the 6th International Thyroid Symposium, Thyroid and Trace Elements, 1996.)

"Resveratrol Induces Apoptosis in Thyroid Cancer Cell Lines via a MAPK– and p53–Dependent Mechanism." *The Journal of Clinical Endocrinology & Metabolism* (Vol 87, No 3) 2002, 1223-32.

Rosen, Irving B., M.D., F.R.C.S.C., F.A.C.S. and Paul Walfish, C.M., M.D., F.R.C.P.C., F.A.C.P., F.R.S.M. "You and Thyroid Cancer." *Thyrobulletin* (Vol 16, No 4) January 1996.

Rosenthal, M. Sara. *50 Ways to Fight Depression without Drugs*. New York: McGraw-Hill, 2002.

Rosenthal, M. Sara. *50 Ways to Prevent and Manage Stress*. New York: McGraw-Hill, 2001.

Rosenthal, M. Sara. *Stopping Cancer at the Source*. Toronto: Your Health Press™, 2001.

Rosenthal, M. Sara. *The Breast Sourcebook*, 2nd edition. New York: McGraw-Hill, 1999.

Rosenthal, M. Sara. *The Hypothyroid Sourcebook*. New York: McGraw-Hill, 2002.

Rosenthal, M. Sara. *The Thyroid Sourcebook,* 4th Edition. New York: McGraw-Hill, 2000.

Rosenthal, M. Sara. *The Thyroid Sourcebook for Women*. New York: McGraw-Hill, 1999.

Rosenthal, M. Sara. *Women Managing Stress*. Toronto: Penguin Books, 2002.

Ross, Douglas S., M.D. "Fine Needle Aspiration Biopsy of Thyroid Nodules." *Thyrobulletin* (Vol 14, No 4) Autumn 1993.

Shmookler, Barry M., M.D. "Errors in Pathology Diagnosis: the Patients' Perspective." Chevy Chase, MD: presented at the Thyroid Cancer Survivor's Annual Conference, September 8, 2000.

Sloca, Paul. "After 14 Years, Nuclear Fallout Study Leads to Questions, Few Answers." *Associated Press*, August 15, 1997. Posted to *www.stardem.com*.

"The Facts about Thyroid Nodules." Daniels Pharmaceuticals, Inc., 1995. (Patient literature.)

Solomon, Diane, M.D. "Fine Needle Aspiration of the Thyroid: an Update." *Thyroid Today* (Vol XVI, No 3) September 1993.

The Thyroid Foundation of America, Inc. "Effects of Thyroxine as Compared with Thyroxine plus Triiodothyronine in Patients with Hypothyroidism." Retrieved online from *www.tsh.org*, February 17, 2000. (Commentary.)

"The Thyroid Foundation of America Suggests More Pregnant Women Be Tested in Response to New Study." Boston, MA: The Thyroid Foundation of America, Inc., August 19, 1999. (Press release.)

"Thyrogen Prescribing Information." Retrieved from *www.genzyme.com*, February 17, 2000.

"Thyroid Cancer Types, Stages and Treatment Overview." Posted to *www.thyca.org*, April 2002.

Toft, Anthony, M.D. "Thyroid Hormone Replacement—One Hormone or Two?" *The New England Journal of Medicine* (Vol 340, No 6) February 11, 1999. (Editorial.)

Utiger, Robert D. "Follow-Up of Patients with Thyroid Carcinoma." *The New England Journal of Medicine* (Vol 337, No 13) September 25, 1997.

Van Middlesworth, L. "Usual and Unusual Isotopes in the Thyroid." Memphis, Tennessee: Department of Physiology, University of Tennessee. (Abstract from the 6th International Thyroid Symposium, Thyroid and Trace Elements, 1996.)

Varl, B., J. Drinovec, and M. Bagar-Posve from the research unit Radenska Redenci, zdravilisko naselje 14, 69252, Radeci, Slovenia. "Iodine Supply with Mineral Water." (Abstract from the 6th International Thyroid Symposium, Thyroid and Trace Elements, 1996.)

Veatch, R.M. "Abandoning Informed Consent." *HCR* (Vol 25 No 2) 1995, 5-12.

Wesche, M.F. et al. "Long-Term Effect of Radioiodine Therapy on Goiter Size in Patients with Non-Toxic Multi-Nodular Goiter." *Clinical Thyroidology* (Vol VIII, Issue 1) January-April 1995.

"Your Hospital Stay." Posted to *www.thyca.org*, April 2002.

Index

ISBN 1553950059-3

9 781553 950592